Home Hospice Navigation

The Caregiver's Guide

Judith R. Sands, RN, MSL, BSN, CCM, CPHRM, CPHQ, LHRM, ARM

Acclaims

For Judith Sands, as for so many of us, all the professional knowledge used daily in her work, took on new significance as she helped her mother through the journey towards the end-of-life. As the challenges became palpable, her new level of understanding leads her to want to help others through the maze of engaging, interacting with, and ultimately being supported by Home Hospice.

The result is a gift to the rest of us - spouses, daughters, sons, and others - who will be called upon to care for those we love on this final journey. In *Home Hospice Navigation*, Ms. Sands assumes the reader is not familiar with the intricacies of the healthcare system related to Hospice. She provides a detailed, yet accessible, description of what the caregiver needs to know to engage supportive care through hospice and to interact with and manage the activities of life as it winds down.

Clearly written, well organized, and comprehensive, this book should be read by anyone who has a loved one with a life-threatening illness or by anyone who wishes to open the end-of-life discussion with their family.

- Geri Amori, PhD, ARM, DFASHRM, CPHRM
Risk Management and Patient Safety Educator and Coach

~

As a healthcare provider and daughter that is going through the caregiving maze, I found Judith's writing on this timely topic of hospice care to be clear, concise and informative, sprinkled with her special warmth and personal antidotes.

- Lisa Feierstein, RN, BSN, MBA
President, Active Healthcare, Inc.

~

This book is a comprehensive roadmap of the many considerations a caregiver must address when a loved one is in decline. It provides clear and straight-forward information as well as helpful links to resources available to assist with many aspects of end-of-life care. I wish I had read it when my parents were in their final years. I highly recommend this book in every respect.

- Jane Green, Caregiver

Contents

Acknowledgments

This book is truly a labor of love, and many people assisted me with this journey. My heartfelt appreciation goes to my personal friends and professional colleagues who provided constant words of support and encouragement that helped keep me going. Your candor and guidance helped shape my vision into a reality.

My appreciation and love to Louis, my husband, editor, and technical support. During mom's decline, he took on many roles including caregiver, mediator, encourager, and all-around supporter.

Foreword

I have been a proud healthcare professional for the past thirty-five years; specifically, a clinical social worker employed as a professional case manager. It is no coincidence that I work in the world of critical illness, for I am the daughter of a physician. During the early phase of my career, I worked with individuals who were diagnosed or living with critical or chronic illnesses. Independent of age or circumstances, the common thread was the challenge for the involved support systems and caregivers to negotiate the progression of illness and implement an appropriate plan-of-care at the end-of-life. The tightrope of balancing communication with respect to individual integrity and the human condition is why the end-of-life processes demand expert attention. Each effort must be carefully orchestrated much like a composer manages the flow and timing of instruments for a symphony.

Of the many knowledge gifts my father passed on to me, one was especially meaningful: to respect the integrity and circumstance of each patient. This was paramount when addressing the end-of-life journey. The five stages of death and dying identified by Elisabeth Kubler Ross in 1969 provide a strong framing for this journey, it remains an emotionally complex one for the majority of people. While I have always found the stages of denial, anger, bargaining, guilt, and acceptance a valuable roadmap of responses for patients and professionals, it is evident that individual coping does not occur sequentially. A patient might start at anger or guilt, as readily as denial. Patients and their families were often at different stages and not on parallel paths. I also witnessed how professionals often struggled with conveying information about prognosis and establishing a definitive plan of care. Providing even the most basic facts around advanced directives could be difficult.

My professional position defined me a large percentage of each day; however, I held another important though more intimate role; that of a daughter who managed a home hospice plan for her father. 2005 was over a decade ago, though it seems like yesterday. My highly respected physician father suffered a series of small vessel strokes, leaving him a far cry from the man I knew. Throughout our journey, my mother would comment "I am grateful for the care we received and appreciate it was so smooth because of who and what you know. But what happens to those who don't have an "Ellen" involved?". My friends still discuss how I "case managed" my father with the same high-quality expectations and fierce advocacy skills I employ for my patients. It is paramount that those in need received the care and comfort deserved at their time of need. It was unacceptable to receive anything less.

My father received home hospice for several months. We were fortunate for having what I would consider a "model" experience. The intake nurse was a colleague, who enveloped me with a hug the size of Texas when she appeared at my parent's apartment for the intake. She took nothing for granted in her initial dialogues with my family, and reminded me how critical it was to check my healthcare professional hat at the door. *"It is time for you to be a daughter. Let us take care of you and your family"*, she said. There was an abundance of clear messaging to both my mother and me during that time, which offered us some control over this very uncontrollable situation.

But what happens to those who don't know anything about hospice, what it offers, and what constitutes a model approach?

In the thirteen years since my father's passing, there has been a tremendous increase in the use of hospice and the resources available to patients and families. In the year 2015, some 1,007,753 Medicare beneficiaries in the United States died under a hospice program. Another 1,381,182 beneficiaries were enrolled in hospice care (National Hospice and Palliative Care Association, 2016).[1] Shared decision making has become the norm for many healthcare organizations. The Internet is a

---

[1] National Hospice and Palliative Care Association (2016) Facts and Figures, Hospice Care in America, National Hospice and Palliative Care Program: Alexandria, VA

hub of resource information, with ample data specific to healthcare and hospice. Social media offers online groups and portals to provide information and support regarding everything from treatment alternatives to funding options. Palliative care is more widely understood and utilized. Society has seen the construct of *end-of-life* evolve to a new framing of *death with dignity*. **Despite the large number and scope of resources available to patients and families, understanding and maneuvering home hospice is misunderstood and often overwhelming.**

Home Hospice Navigation: The Caregiver's Guide provides an organized and comprehensive roadmap to understand better the key areas needed for a quality home hospice experience. Judith Sands, an experienced nurse, case manager, and patient safety professional, uses her journey with her mother to offer a necessary and valuable tool for patients and caregivers. It guides them down the often-complex hospice path, providing foundational knowledge and pertinent resources. The book is intentional in its design, organizing the diverse and robust content in a logical order. There are concrete discussions on the multiple types of documents used in advanced care planning (e.g., advanced directives, POLST) and levels of hospice care. There is crucial content on the misconceptions of hospice, which is a must for caregivers to know. The information on the various types of caregiving and chapter on 'Helpful Hints' found me remembering so many questions that I, an experienced healthcare professional had going through the process. The appendices are chock full of practical templates to organize the experience, from medication to life management. Resources referenced in the book are available on the website www.JudithSands.com.

The book is an equally integral resource for healthcare professionals who work with hospice patients and their caregivers. This book is especially meaningful in the education and mentoring of students and more seasoned professionals across the healthcare industry. It provides a critical lens to view the distinct world of those involved with home hospice: one often fraught with indecision, fear, and anxiety of what is to come. It offers strong content to promote greater awareness for persons coping with their end-of-life; one of the most vulnerable times of the life course. The themes are universal and resonate with all patients, practitioners, providers, and personal caregivers, alike. The book empowers the ethical mantras mandated by all healthcare professionals of patient fidelity, integrity, and individuality; my father would have approved.

Ellen Fink-Samnick MSW, ACSW, LCSW, CCM, CRP
Principal, EFS Supervision Strategies, LLC

A Tribute to Mom

Not enough can be s~
of valor who wou
her many special a
avoiding the limelight a

know?" The truth was ~
picked it up on her wa
to Buffalo.

Mom was born in Liver,
haired baby; a fourth child c
emigrated separately from Russia
Abraham had rented a room from Ru
rest was history. Baby Anita was doted or,
were in their teens when she arrived.

One of the "s~
as the "family a
goods still have
was a "better
marriage she
dessert firs
be great.

During WWII, she lived with her sister in Irela,
end and the family was reestablishing themselv
Liverpool, Grandpa believed it was time to get mom n
saw some of the prospects and decided she was not havin,
She made the declaration that she was going off to India, to se
could do it make it a "better place." There was a standor,
compromise was that mom could go to Canada. After working in a v
end dress shop, and then managing a day camp at a hotel in th
Laurentian Mountains, she was set up on a blind date with my father,
Henry. Dad, an avid skier, came to the hotel for the weekend. Mom was
not particularly pleased about being "set up." She manipulated the
situation; and used the date as the opportunity to dine at one of
Montreal's most exclusive and expensive restaurants. She suggested
Ruby Fu, a Chinese establishment. I still wonder how she pulled this off
since neither mom nor dad was a big fan of Chinese food until much later
in life. It must have been "ordained!"

Mom could never lie. On another of dad's visits to see her before the
wedding, mom had dad over for dinner. My dad, the jokester and king of
the backhanded compliments, told her the "meal was so good you could
not have made it." Mom, crestfallen turned to him and said, "how did you

hat her friend Dorie made the dinner for her, mom
y home from work. After the wedding, mom moved

ills" she picked was the recipe for what is now known
pple cake." This cake and many of mom's other baked
a strong following. She was affectionately told that she
baker than a cook." Mom shared that in her early days of
worked the menu backward. She always started making the
t, figuring if dinner was no good, then at least dessert would

m loved to shop, and never turned down a mall or outlet shopping
en if she did not like the latest styles. She was excited and was
s ready for the 5 a.m. Black Friday sales, even if it meant driving
ss town to stand in line to be among the first admitted.

Mom has often said that the last third of her life was her best. She
was blessed with two grandchildren, and wonderful in-laws with whom
she traveled to China, India, and Russia. The lunch dates with Dorothy
(my mother-in-law) were legendary; often going for a burger and onion
rings, and agreeing that they had the best set of grandsons.

Nana, as she was known to my boys, was very doting. She made all
the boys' baby food that was affectionately known as "Nana food,"
babysitting, picking the kids up from daycare and school, taking them to
doctor appointments, and being present at school events. Although the
boys were challenging at times, especially when they were young, she
loved taking them out for lunch, only to be amazed at the volume of food
that could be consumed. Mom made noddle pudding by the pan load and
was admonished for pre-cutting any baked goods, since the dainty
portion size she was accustomed to serving, was not in keeping with the
portion size of growing boys. She often reflected on the wonderful trip
we had taken with the boys to London, she finally got to play tourist and
visit all the sights that she wanted to see.

No matter where mom lived if any of her friends or those in need were ill or needed a meal, she was the first in line to assist. Her endless energy, compassion, and love for others were her hallmark.

Mom developed a deep affection for her grandson's high school friends who treated her with the utmost of respect and helped her, while she "supervised" in our absence. One of the skills that she acquired was "beer pong," yet I doubt she actually drank any beer. I am still waiting to find out if she was given her beverage of choice, gin.

Mom was excited when we shared that we were moving to Raleigh, she advised that she was up for the challenge. Mom was eager to move into her own place, a newly built independent living complex. She was known as one of the five "Golden Girls." The five ladies were all new residents, they met daily at 5 p.m. for wine, and each brought some snacks. They looked out for each other, and they had a very special relationship, mom was the last surviving member of that original group. Over the years she made many very special friends who have been wonderful at socializing and visiting her, keeping her spirits high. When her health started to decline and limited her mobility, she often commented on how surprised she was at the number of people that kept coming in to check on her and visit with her.

It will never be forgotten that mom always puts others before herself. She was a committed peacemaker who wanted the family, her community, and the world to be a better place. Mom was a role model, mentor, coach, guide, and friend to many. You will not be forgotten. You have touched the hearts of many, and you are cherished.

The Book's Evolution

As a respected healthcare professional with expertise in care coordination and discharge planning, nothing could have prepared me for having to take on the responsibilities for managing mom's care, especially in the home hospice setting. Throughout my professional career, I have sat with families discussing how the individual and family wanted to approach end-of-life care. During these sessions, options to meet the individual's wishes often included the discussion about hospice and the most appropriate setting for such care.

Over the years, I encountered the hospice benefit first hand, my father died in a hospice house, my mother-in-law was on home hospice, and when faced with my mother's declining health, she elected home hospice care. We were fortunate that we had the difficult discussions when she was in good health and could articulate and share her wishes, revise her will, update her Advance Directive and name her healthcare surrogates; those individuals who could make healthcare decisions when she was incapable.

Mom, a very special unassuming individual who always implicitly trusted the medical profession, did not believe in human suffering or prolonging the dying process. Over the years she had seen just about all of her friends and loved one's pass, continually expressing her wish not to have a prolonged and painful death. Being an only child, who had always been close to mom, her wishes were known and were in alignment with my beliefs. Mom, a very private individual was not one to acknowledge or share that her health was declining. Although we lived a mile apart, and saw each other daily, she was a master at concealing her health issues. One of the key issues impacting her ability to maintain independence was her slips and falls. In fact, at her surprise 94th birthday party, the surprise was on us; she avoided sharing that she had fallen, was in pain and unable to walk. We carried her to the party and the next day she enrolled in home hospice, in keeping with her wishes.

Role reversals become common at this stage; either a spouse who was cared for by that individual assumes new responsibilities, or children are stepping into the caregiving and decision-making roles. Depending on the individual and respective caregiver, this can be very traumatic and unsettling. This may be the time you elect to hire a professional care manager to oversee the day-to-day issues of care coordination and management. What you should remember is that you have options.

As you read this book, remember that it is written primarily for the caregiver. This may be you, or someone sharing the journey with you. Your loved one is an integral part of the decision process and should have significant input on their care management. If they are not able to participate, you should try to honor their end-of-life wishes. Everyone's situation is a little different, yet there are many commonalities, and through different experiences, best practices and approaches are identified. These are being made available to assist you in the caregiving role. Navigating home hospice is not prescriptive; there is no one-size-fits-all formula. You have to find what works for you. You should feel empowered to ask for what you need and slow to accept "no" as an answer. The book's glossary can help you understand unfamiliar terms. Know that you are not alone and that you will learn a lot about yourself, your loved one, friends and family during your journey.

Disclaimer

There may be state and insurance coverage variations. This book is a general guide and not intended as specific advice or medical advice.

How to Read this Book

Throughout the book, you will see informational icons:

 Helps you identify import considerations

 A personal note

 A link to this resource can be found on www.JudithSands.com

Introduction

Having to acknowledge the agonizing and gut-wrenching reality that pain, symptom management, and suffering have taken over your loved one's daily routine is a very upsetting realization. You may not have seen it coming, and it will hit you like a freight train. Watching your loved one's focus shift from the ability to carry out activities of daily living, plan pleasurable activities, and enjoyable events; to stressing on how to get through the next few hours. The awareness that medical management no longer can provide a cure is a hard realization for many to accept. The conversation that you should have with your loved one may be distressing. Speaking openly of mortality with your loved one may be very difficult or avoided. Some cultures and families try to shield the individual from the reality of death or the lack of a cure; often it is the fear of losing hope. It is common to hear a family say, "dad is not dying in the next week, so he doesn't need hospice." Hospice is another level of care that is available for pain and symptom management. This topic will be discussed later in the book. For now, recognize that not utilizing hospice, means that you may miss the opportunity for better symptom management and the opportunity for your loved one to get their affairs in order. Not leveraging hospice services can add a burden to your family. In these situations, it is often helpful for the primary message to be one focused on managing the symptoms (pain, shortness of breath, nausea, etc.) and being kept comfortable.

Hospice services provide a unique combination of clinical and psychological services to individuals with a diagnosis of terminal illness or a failure to thrive (calorie or protein malnutrition), and a life expectancy of less than six months. Unfortunately, a common misconception is that hospice is euthanasia, mercy killing or assisted suicide (the practice of intentionally hastening or ending life to relieve pain and suffering). Hospice providers (certain home health agencies with a hospice program or dedicated hospice providers) are committed to assisting those nearing the end-of-life, restoring dignity, and providing a sense of personal fulfillment. Hospice should be thought of as living fully as long as possible and helping your loved one to die a peaceful and comfortable death.

Deciding to explore hospice care and learning of the option to obtain better pain and symptom management can be a liberating experience for you and the family. It is a journey that you will not have to travel alone. A team of professionals will customize a plan of care, with emphasis on keeping your loved one comfortable and providing emotional and spiritual support (if desired) to everyone. You, the caregiver, play a critical and valuable role, and also need to feel supported and cherished.

The role of caregiver has been increasingly recognized as an important one. A caregiver can be a relative, partner, friend, neighbor, or a person contracted from an agency which provides a broad range of assistance. Care functions can vary widely based on your loved one's needs, and what you are able and willing to handle.

This book is designed to be practical, help set expectations, and guide you through the conversation with the attending physician, hospice representatives, family members, and loved ones. You are not the first or the last person having to deal with making the difficult decisions about the type of care to be provided during this challenging time. Take advantage of the information and resources being shared. Begin conversations with your loved one about how they would like to spend the final phase of life, and what is necessary to achieve those wishes. Share this information with others. Utilize the information to become knowledgeable about options, stay organized, and recharged while caregiving.

Twilight of Life

Until the mid-20th century, dying was viewed as a natural progression; a loved one died surrounded by family, community members, and religious leaders in their homes. Often, they were the center of attention and most people had contact with the dying. How death was viewed changed when the dying process shifted to hospitals or nursing homes where medicines and medical equipment could prolong the dying; loved ones were isolated, and visitors tended to stay away. The change in death location resulted in many individuals becoming inexperienced and uncomfortable with dying since it was distanced care, and "out-of-sight."

Palliative care is the term used by healthcare professionals to indicate a level of care that focuses on symptom relief for individuals with serious illnesses. Typically, those who take advantage of palliative care are still undergoing aggressive or curative therapies that may include: dialysis, chemotherapy or radiation. The palliative care team is specially trained to work with the loved one, providing an extra level of clinical, emotional and spiritual support to manage symptoms. Palliative care is a level of care and is often used as "pre-hospice" care; a beneficial symptom management approach since they are still receiving active treatment. The key phrase is "still receiving active treatment." Once your loved one stops receiving active treatment, they can transition to the next level of care, hospice.

Hospice specializes in the caring for the terminally ill or those with a "failure to thrive." The medical community describes the failure to thrive as the gradual decline in health that may be associated with chronic disease, characterized by weight loss, decreased appetite, poor nutrition and physical inactivity. A person with "failure to thrive" may also have dehydration, depression, and immune deficiency. Hospice provides a well-coordinated, proactive, supportive team that not only tends to your loved one, but also to the caregivers. Determining the extent of care, necessary comfort measures, and where the care will be provided are questions for consideration. Here is the dilemma many people face; when you are healthy, the family does not want to have the uncomfortable end-of-life discussion. When you must have the discussion, it is already very stressful, and decision making can become clouded with emotion. It is best to have end-of-life discussions before hospice services are needed, and the stress of the situation is upon you.

Advance Care Planning: End-of-Life Discussions

End-of-life planning is not something you have to do alone. Since January 1, 2016, physicians are more motivated to discuss Advance Care Planning with Medicare beneficiaries during the Annual Wellness Visit (AWV). Why? Follow the money trail - physicians can now bill for this valuable face-to-face Advance Directive discussion, with or without completing relevant legal forms. Medicare views Advance Care Planning as a preventative health service, so deductibles and coinsurances are waived for this discussion; eliminating cost as a barrier to this important discussion. Counseling provides the opportunity to help your loved one express their wishes about future treatments.

Everyone can take advantage of the Institute for Healthcare Improvement's step by step Conversation Starter Kit to assist in identifying and sharing what matters in end-of-life care. This resource assists in guiding the conversation relating to care and treatment wishes, level of involvement by family or caregivers, sharing of information and preferences. It walks you through the discussion process and provides a tool for documenting a shared understanding of what matters most to the individual and their loved ones. The Conversation Starter Kit is in numerous languages and is free.

There are several documents (collectively known as Advance Directives). The three forms comprising the Advance Directives include a Living Will, Physician Order for Life-Sustaining Treatment (POLST), also known as Medical Orders for Life-Sustaining Treatment (MOLST), or a Do Not Resuscitate (DNR)/Do Not Attempt Resuscitation (DNAR) form, and Durable Power of Attorney for Healthcare Decisions. Everyone should have these documents on record, even if you are healthy. Hospice will ask you to complete the DNR/DNAR before admission. POLST summarizes your loved one's wishes in the form of a medical order set. POLST does not replace the DNR/DNAR, and its requirement varies by state.

Living Will

The Five Wishes, developed by Aging with Dignity, is one of the popular living wills. It is written in everyday language and helps guide the conversation about care in times of serious illness. It has been used by more than 19 million individuals and is available in 28 different languages. The Five Wishes are:

- "The Person I Want to Make Health Care Decisions for Me When I Can't"
- "The Kind of Medical Treatment I Want or Don't Want"
- "How Comfortable I Want to Be"
- "How I Want People to Treat Me"
- "What I Want My Loved Ones to Know"

Each of the "Wishes" has clarifying statements to help the individual to determine, state, and share their end-of-life care wishes.

Five Wishes online allows on-screen completion and can then be printed. It can be ordered from the association for a modest charge. Some hospitals and healthcare organizations also make this resource available to individuals at no charge. Copies should be provided to the family physician, family members, and included with the Advance Directives. ✎

Physician Order for Life-Sustaining Treatment (POLST)/ Medical Orders for Life-Sustaining Treatment (MOLST)

Another legal document is the Physician Order for Life-Sustaining Treatment (POLST). It is a set of standing medical orders, based on informed and shared decision making, that accompanies your loved one to any care setting. The intent is to define the values, beliefs, religious views and goals for desired end-of-life care. It identifies the treatments that your loved one does and does not want; recognizing that natural death is not the same as killing. POLST does not allow for active

6

euthanasia or physician-assisted suicide. The complete list of electronic POLST registries can be located online. ✍

DNR/DNAR

The Do Not Resuscitate (DNR)/Do Not Attempt Resuscitation (DNAR) documents the end-of-life discussion made with a physician, and a medical order is written instructing healthcare providers and caregivers not to attempt cardiopulmonary resuscitation (CPR) in the event of cardiac or respiratory arrest (heart or breathing stops). With a valid DNR order on record, your loved one will not be given CPR under these circumstances. Although the DNR order is written at the request of your loved one, or their healthcare surrogate, it must be signed by a physician to be valid. A non-hospital DNR order is written for individuals who are at home and do not want to receive CPR. That document must be readily available, often kept on the refrigerator or bedside table.

Durable Power of Attorney

A durable power of attorney (POA) gives someone the power to act in your loved one's place to handle specific health, legal and financial responsibilities should they ever become mentally incapacitated. There are two types of durable powers of attorney: POA for healthcare and POA for finances. POA for healthcare gives a designated person the authority to make health care decisions on behalf of someone. POA for finances gives a designated person the authority to make legal or financial decisions for someone. The POA responsibilities for healthcare and financial decision making may be assigned to one or two separate individuals.

Did you know that in some states, a court-appointed guardian makes end-of-life decisions in the absence of an Advance Directive? If you do not want a stranger making end-of-life decisions for your loved one, then you need to have an Advance Directive. Ensure that your loved one's healthcare decisions are being made by the person they want. Get a POA!

Healthcare Surrogate

Typically, within the circle of care, one individual tends to be the spokesperson and advocates for your loved one. This person is known as the healthcare surrogate. The healthcare surrogate is appointed by your loved one, in writing, through a Living Will, or a Power of Attorney (POA). The individual may be entrusted with either healthcare, financial or both responsibilities. **POA authority stops at the time of death**. The financial implication is that if you need money from your loved one's account to pay bills, you may not have access to their bank account until after the estate is probated. Depending on the individual's status at the time they enter hospice, you may or may not have sufficient time to modify and change some of the financial documents to include a POA or co-trustee. Consult your financial planner, banker, and attorney to discuss, review and determine what actions are needed for your particular situation. Documentation requirements vary by state and typically can be completed without an attorney. The formally assigned role of healthcare surrogate is designed to ensure that your loved ones' wishes and interests are protected. It may also be a designated paid professional (care coordinator) or an informally assigned role given the individual's background, education, experiences or temperament. The healthcare surrogate is the person who helps ensure that needs are being addressed quickly and appropriately. This individual should be named on Privacy Notices as the individual with whom medical information may be discussed. Remember to inform the person that has been designated as the healthcare surrogate.

There are times when the healthcare surrogate may feel like the "wicked witch of the west," yet there must be someone who is the "glue" for the circle of care team members. The healthcare surrogate stays on top of the care planning and delivery process, speaks out when things are not going well, and alerts the team to concerning issues. They escalate concerns when a Certified Nursing Assistant (CNA) or nurse does not arrive as expected and holds people accountable for supplies and medication orders that are not correct or have not been delivered as promised. Having that designated spokesperson helps ensure that there is one individual who is managing and orchestrating on behalf of the loved one. It is also helpful that caregivers and members of the hospice team have only one or two people with whom they communicate. It is unrealistic to expect them to speak with multiple individuals. The Institute for Healthcare Improvement has a free downloadable resource titled How to Choose a Health Care Proxy & How to Be a Health Care Proxy. It is a valuable tool for role responsibility and clarification. These excellent resources will assist you and your loved one in choosing the appropriate healthcare proxy and understanding the responsibilities of the role. ✎

Hospice Misconceptions

There are many misconceptions about hospice. Here are a few of the more common ones.

- **Hospice is a place to go and die**. Hospice is designed for an individual with life-limiting illness in need of symptom control and comfort. Hospice services may be provided where they live, and the location of care may change as their condition changes. The care supports the loved one and family. Choosing hospice is not a death sentence, rather a service for comfort care and symptom management.

- **Hospice care is expensive**. Medicare, Medicaid, and most insurance plans cover hospice services. Uninsured individuals can often qualify for services under individual hospice compassion programs. Lack of insurance or sound finances should NOT be a barrier to obtaining hospice services.

- **Morphine will speed up the dying process or kill my loved one**. Morphine Sulfate is an opium derivative, especially effective at controlling pain and reducing the symptoms of shortness of breath. Although highly addictive, it is a very effective medication providing comfort to hospice individuals. So, how much is too much? As a generalized reference point, hospice may start oral morphine at 0.25 mg or 0.50 mg. A lethal dose of morphine could be anywhere between 60-200 mg (depending on many factors).

- **Hospice is only for cancer or AIDS patients**. Hospice services are available for a variety of diagnoses beyond cancer and AIDS, including: Congestive Heart Failure (CHF), end-stage kidney disease, failure to thrive (calorie or protein malnutrition), Parkinson's, and Alzheimer's. There are medically accepted criteria for admission into hospice and individuals are evaluated based on their condition.

- **Once in hospice, there is no getting out of the program**. An individual may disenroll at any time from the hospice service. If they want to re-enroll in the future, there may be a waiting period set by Medicare, Medicaid, and various insurance regulations.

Home Hospice Navigation

- **Hospice care requires the individual to stop taking medication.** Hospice focuses on symptom relief rather than a curative approach. All medications are reviewed for intended use and effectiveness, along with any unique issues. Chemotherapy and radiation therapy are typically stopped in hospice.
- **Hospice always sedates to control pain.** Many people fear pain more than the dying process. Management of pain typically begins with the lowest possible dose to control symptoms. Over time there may be sedation; the goal is to keep your loved one comfortable.

When to Consider Hospice Services

Loved ones are encouraged to ask about the possibility of hospice appropriateness. This is another way of discussing and clarifying Advance Directives and presenting information on hospice services. Although hospice services may not be appropriate or selected at this time, it plants the idea for the future. Hospice care is typically for people with a life expectancy of six months or less. Hospice services may be extended by the hospice medical director, or another hospice physician recertifies the terminal illness of life expectancy of six months or less. Don't let the definitions scare or deter you from obtaining the best care for your loved one. Mom was in hospice for 11 months. She wanted to be as comfortable as possible and utilized the services available to her.

When you are in a hospital or under the care of a physician for an *active medical condition* you expect to be offered treatment options. Hospice care is often the forgotten option since your loved one is no longer receiving treatment for an active medical condition. To assist with deciding when to ask for hospice services, consider these questions:

- Despite good medical care, do symptoms progress to the point where relief cannot be adequately obtained?
- There have been multiple hospitalizations, emergency department visits, or frequent use of other healthcare services?
- Physician or specialist have said, "there is nothing more that can be done to slow or cure the condition"?
- Do the side effects of medical treatments outweigh the benefits?

If any of these questions are answered "yes," then there is a good chance that hospice services may be an appropriate continuing care option. **Hospice services do not hasten the dying process**. Hospice care is focused on comfort and symptom management, and easing the dying process. Hospice services and interventions tend to be intense at the period of enrollment when care is being initiated and coordinated between the various hospice team members; during a significant change in a loved one's condition; and near the time of death when additional care and services may be needed.

Hospice appropriateness is based on medical criteria and guidelines that are condition specific. The individual's appropriateness for hospice care is determined by the physician. Frequently, the attending physician is the one to suggest hospice services, but not always. Some physicians delay or do not think to offer the hospice option; that does not mean that hospice care may not be beneficial. It is perfectly appropriate to raise the question directly and ask "Is hospice care appropriate at this time?"

The Case for Hospice

Situation #1: a non-cancer diagnosis

John is 75 years old, has end-stage cardiomyopathy (advanced heart disease), a pacemaker for nine years, is 5'8" and weighs 80lb. He is dependent on oxygen most of the time. His feet are swollen, especially if they have not been on the elevated wheelchair footrest, activities outside the home are very limited. Lately, John's appetite has decreased, he is losing interest in food, and he does not want to go through a pacemaker battery replacement. His wife is doing more of his personal care and is becoming overwhelmed.

What are the considerations?

- Has John made his wishes known?
- Does John have an Advance Directive?
- Has John said anything about his quality of life and his wishes for the future?

Actions to consider:

- Consider speaking to the primary care physician and/or cardiologist (heart doctor) about how they view his future
- Ask the medical team about appropriateness for hospice

- Ask for a hospice evaluation to learn more about the program and how they can help

Situation #2: a cancer diagnosis

Mary is 45, with stage 4 breast cancer; she has been fighting the disease with surgery and chemotherapy for the last five years. At this point, there is no cure for Mary's condition. Her pain is not well managed, and she is suffering from several side effects. She is not able to participate in doing the activities that have brought her joy in the past. Mary shared that she wants some control over her life.

What are the considerations?

- Has Mary made hers wishes known?
- Does Mary have an Advance Directive?
- Has Mary said anything about her quality of life and her wishes for the future?

Actions to consider:

- Consider speaking to the primary care physician and/or oncologist (cancer doctor) about how they view her future
- Ask the medical team about appropriateness for hospice
- Ask for a hospice evaluation to learn more about the program and how they can help

How to Involve Hospice

You can call a hospice provider for a free evaluation of hospice appropriateness. The conversation can take place even if hospice options have not been discussed with a physician, or you are curious about available options. Should hospice be appropriate, the hospice provider can help you, and your loved one have the conversation with your physician. Hospice is easy to work with, and there is no pressure. Your situation may indicate that at the current time hospice is not appropriate, but at some future point conditions may change and hospice will be appropriate.

Hospice Conversation

The conversation with hospice should take place in a quiet location with minimal disruptions. Allow sufficient time for the discussion about your loved one's condition, the hospice program, indicated hospice services, and the development of a Plan of Care matching your loved one's wishes. Time must be provided to fully express wishes and preferences, ensuring that they are in keeping with the hospice program.

Making the big decision to take advantage of hospice services should not be a dreaded one. While it can be emotionally difficult; for many, it is a natural progression based on Advance Care Planning. It is the next step in open communication for sharing spiritual and medical values, treatment or management goals and wishes with the physician and family. These wishes are ideally documented in an Advance Directive or shared orally, and help to formulate the care and treatment plan as the individual enters the last phase of life. Dying is part of the cycle of life. With the increasing use of medical technology, the dying process is often extended; changing where and how people experience dying. For many, making this decision means they have more control over how they are living. It is the recognition that the quality of living is most important and aggressive treatment is no longer going to improve life. Often the side effects of treatment make the living process very uncomfortable.

Hospice helps terminally ill individuals live comfortably; it is not just for individuals with cancer. Individuals with other end-stage conditions and symptoms may benefit. Conditions may include:

- Failure to thrive (frail with significant weight loss)
- Parkinson's or neurological disease (stroke and coma)
- AIDS
- Pain management
- Difficulty with bodily functions and movement
- Dependence on others for feeding, bathing, toileting, dressing, and transfers

- Advanced heart, liver, kidney, or lung disease

- Difficulty with nausea & vomiting

- Changing or decreasing level of consciousness

- Alzheimer's and dementia

The focus of the hospice care is on pain and symptom management; keeping your loved one comfortable. The decision to sign up for hospice services is ideally made with sufficient lead time so that the many hospice services and benefits can be taken advantage of early on, not just the final phase of pain and symptom management. A DNR/DNAR form (a hospice requirement) must be available before the admission process to enter a hospice program is completed. The DNR/DNAR form is the acknowledgment that aggressive medical interventions (intubation – breathing tube, Cardio Pulmonary Resuscitation (CPR) and artificial nutrition) will not take place. Every effort will be made to keep your loved one comfortable and not to speed up the dying process.

Personal Note: I find that humor brings a certain level of levity to a serious situation. While managing my mother's care, I received a call from an elderly caregiver who was challenged about how to manage the declining status of her husband. He had undergone several hospital admissions; was not able to take advantage of rehabilitation; unable to take care of himself; and was very demanding. She had heard about hospice and was curious about the benefits package. During the conversation, she was extremely agitated and often referred to the benefits program as "hostage care." That term has stuck with me. My mom and I laughed about it all the time. Despite the humor, please remember that no one is ever a hostage in hospice.

Patient Choice

There are choices and options as to which hospice agency will provide the hospice service. Medicare beneficiaries must be provided with a list of Medicare-approved hospice providers, and your loved one can choose the hospice agency of their choice to provide services. If your loved one is not a Medicare beneficiary, then Medicaid or the insurance company will typically provide a list of approved hospices. We all want to believe that the people we trust with our care will always look out for us. Most of the time this is true; however, there are cases where a physician may specify a hospice entity that may truly not be the best option for your loved one. Speak to your physician, case manager, family, and friends to learn about their experiences with different hospice agencies. It may be advisable to ask the physician if they have any management or Board role with a particular hospice. Unfortunately, sometimes geographic location may limit the number of available hospice provider choices.

 Be sure to ask the physician if they are willing to work with the hospice staff on managing care. Either way, hospice has physicians who will direct and manage care.

Not All Hospices Are Created Equal

When enrolling in hospice, it is the time when certain medical treatments and services may be discontinued, with the shift in focus from curative (active treatment) to comfort management. Some hospices are non-profit entities while others are for-profit, the difference in ownership may affect individual care and the number of services available. When speaking with the hospice representative, ask about the number of individuals who elect to discontinue hospice services from this agency (disenrollment rate). Currently, this data is not published, yet it will give you an indication of how other users of a particular hospice perceive their level of satisfaction. What you are looking for is an understanding of how care is provided.

It is worth noting that not all hospices are created equal. All hospices provide a core set of services. The spectrum of hospice services differs between hospice agencies, and they can vary by state, county, and even within cities. In some cases, it is a home care agency that has a program focused on providing in-home hospice services. The home care agency may not have the ability to easily transition or move the individual to an in-patient hospice facility, should there be a change in condition or they are no longer able to be managed at home. Other hospice entities have a full spectrum of services and can help with moving the person as care needs change. An important topic you should inquire about is staffing and backup assistance, especially when care is provided at home. Perception of a hospice's level of care and service is often judged by the relationship with a particular nurse or CNA that usually provides care. You will want to understand if are they currently understaffed, and how they address the situation when someone calls in sick or goes on vacation. How will your loved one's routine be disrupted?

You may think the hospice financial status (for-profit vs. not-for-profit) is not your relevant; however, it may impact the range of services you receive. The message to you is, understand the value each hospice organization can bring to your situation. Research has shown that given the financial reimbursement models for hospice services, the costs of care are higher during the enrollment period, during a major change in condition, and close to the time of death. The vast majority of individuals in hospice are Medicare beneficiaries. As such, the reimbursement model is critical to the financial survival of the hospice and impacts the quality and amount of care delivered to the individual. Medicare pays a fixed daily dollar amount to hospice for each individual served. Given the tax consequences of for-profit and not-for-profit status; for-profit hospices tend to do more community resource work and set up foundations. Foundations typically use the funds to support community outreach and assist individuals with care related expenses and crisis funding (heating and cooling bills, small household repairs and travel for visitors).

There should not be a difference in the quality of care you receive if the hospice used is a for-profit or a non-profit agency, but sometimes it does occur. The regulations are the same; all licensed and certified hospices must comply with State law and Federal Regulations governing hospice care. In any field of business, there are the "good," and the "bad," and hospice is no different. Non-profit organizations, including non-profit hospices, do not pay federal, state, or local taxes. The major difference between for-profit and non-profit hospice is that a non-profit organization is not allowed to show a profit at the end of their financial year. Should a non-profit organization have a profit, it can use their discretion in spending that money. Many non-profit hospices will use extra funds for fundraising events or provide donations to special programs within their community. All hospices are paid on a per-diem basis for every day the patient is enrolled in the program. Those hospices that "skimp" on services can increase their profits at the expense of the patients and families.

For-profit hospices typically have a higher proportion of individuals in nursing homes and a lower proportion of individuals living at home. Individuals in nursing homes often cost hospice agencies less money over time, since the facility staff is providing most of the direct care. Enrolling in a non-profit may lower the risk of fewer nursing visits and be less likely to receive more intense levels of care for loved ones undergoing a crisis in their symptoms. Some research studies have revealed that more patients were being discharged from for-profit hospices close to the time of death. One of the best indicators of whether or not you should choose one hospice or another is the direct personal reference from someone you know and trust who has had recent experience with the hospice services.

The Centers for Medicare & Medicaid Services released Hospice Compare in August 2017. ✑ This is a website that lets the user compare up to three hospice agencies at a time, among 3,876 nationwide that were available at website inception. Through the website, individuals can compare how hospice entities performed in seven categories (Individual preferences and Managing pain and treating symptoms), including screening for pain and breathing difficulties, and how many individuals on opioids were offered treatment for constipation. Searches can be done by either searching a particular provider or hospice entities by location. It is important to recognize that the measures are based on self-reporting by hospices, and should not be the only basis for selecting a particular hospice provider. Family ratings of hospices have recently been added.

For-Profit and Non-profit Hospices ✎

National Hospice Survey Results, For-Profit Status, Community Engagement, and Service ✎

How For-Profit Hospices Compare to Non-profit Hospices ✎

Differences in Care at For-Profit Hospices ✎

Profit vs. Non-Profit Hospice ... Is There a Difference? ✎

Starting Hospice Benefits

Communication and asking questions is key to a successful hospice experience. Do not hesitate to share your concerns with the hospice nurse. Medicare hospice care is given in benefit periods. Hospice care follows Medicare payment rules. When you hear about 90-day and 60-day certification periods, these are directly related to payment rules for hospice reimbursement. Hospice care is provided for two 90-day periods followed by an unlimited number of 60-day periods, with the appropriate physician recertification. This physician certification is based on the individual's medical status. Commercial payors also require physician certification based on the individual's medical status.

The Admission Process

The hospice admission process takes time and involves several hospice representatives. Typically, it begins with an admission nurse; this process may take one to two hours depending on your familiarity with hospice services, clarification of wishes, the medical condition, and determining the services and equipment that will be needed. Medications and therapies will be reviewed, and determinations may be made as to discontinuation of existing services (such as physical therapy), and what equipment and comfort measures are needed. Admission will set in motion the delivery of needed equipment such as a hospital bed, over-bed table, oxygen, or wheelchair. Over time, different equipment may be added. Equipment that is no longer used will be removed from the home.

After-hours, weekend, holiday and admissions

The hospice admission process can take place during non-business hours. Often the process takes longer due to physician availability for treatment orders, reduced hospice and supply vendor staffing. Be patient, yet stay in contact with the hospice on-call nurse to ensure that you have a time frame as to when the appointment to sign the required admission documents and assessment of your loved one will take place. The identification of care needs and starting the process to obtain the immediately needed medications and services will take place during this appointment. Additionally, the hospice will make delivery arrangements.

The hospice parade

The nurse, social worker, clergy, and dietician will initiate contact after the admission process has been completed. Often each of these specialists makes their own appointment to meet with you and your loved one. These visits take time, so ask if they can make a joint (combined) visit, thus information is not being repeated, and it helps to start forming the care team, facilitating quicker resolution of care issues. Depending on needs, follow-up appointments may be scheduled every few days, weekly, or every two weeks. Be sure to let the hospice professional know if you need a change in visit frequency or feel overwhelmed by the number of different individuals involved in the care. Do not be afraid to discuss the role and purpose of the various representatives and their interventions; at times, it may feel overwhelming. These professionals should be providing assistance and support.

Personal Note: Mom was not receptive to the assistance of the social worker. After several visits, mom requested that she no longer visit. I kept the lines of communication open, should her professional expertise be needed at a later date.

Change in where hospice services are being provided

When a person on hospice moves from their home to an alternative location such as an assisted living facility (ALF), nursing home, or hospice facility, there is a new intake process.

Be prepared to answer the new set of intake questions; specifically, what is prompting the change in care location. You may ask yourself "I've already answered these questions! Can't they read the paperwork?" The reason for the repetition is that there are cases where mistakes have been made in transcription or clarification is needed. This approach helps ensure that any errors/confusion are identified and corrected. Once moved out of the home and into an alternative care setting, typically the amount of direct physical care given by the circle of care tends to decrease. The various staff members at the facilities then become more involved with care coordination and supply management. Placement takes away some of the direct care and management burdens for caregivers. Caregivers are no longer responsible for direct care, medications, supplies, and meal preparation.

Contact information – keep track of the actual hospice team members working with you and when visits are planned.

- Hospice Name and Contact information
- Registered Nurse (RN)
- Advanced Registered Nurse Practitioner (APRN)

- Aide/CNA
- Social Worker
- Spiritual Care
- Other

Your loved one's medical status will determine the frequency of visits by the hospice team members; for many families, the RN and the CNA are often the most frequently encountered people and the face of hospice care. Visits to the primary care physician may be in order if the medical condition has not deteriorated too much, and the ability to walk or be transported is viable. In this case, the hospice physician is still involved, but behind the scene. If your loved one is less mobile or in a facility, then the hospice physician is probably the one to visit and examine them. One thing to realize is that the physician may be on rotation and the same physician may not be seeing your loved one in the future. The lack of continuity by a single physician may be an issue at times, but it can be well managed with good communication.

Transfer or Change in Hospice Providers

Should the decision be made to change hospice providers, how is this done, so benefits are not lost? Once in each election period, a change can be made to a different hospice provider. Your loved one must file with the hospice from which they are receiving care and with the newly designated hospice. If the decision is made to change hospice providers, it should be done with due diligence and thought. Continuity of care is paramount, and you will need to work with both agencies during the transition.

Centers for Medicare & Medicaid Services – Medicare Hospice Benefits ✎

Medicare & Hospice Benefits – Getting Started – Care & support for people who are terminally ill ✎

Considerations:

- Involve your loved one as much as possible, or as much as they wish to be involved, in the care coordination and hospice process
- Know who has been designated the healthcare proxy. Is this person serving as the designated spokesperson?
  - Are there individuals in the circle of care who are opposed to hospice?
  - Are there individuals in the circle of care who are opposed to the healthcare proxy?
  - Is the healthcare proxy in close geographical proximity to the individual to facilitate the timely signing of legal and medical documents?
- Will there be legal, medical or religious representatives included in care planning?

- Copies of Advance Directives (Living Wills, DNR/DNAR, or Durable Power of Attorney for Healthcare Decisions) should be kept readily available in the home and not stored in safe-deposit boxes. Copies should be given to physicians, local hospitals, independent and Assisted Living Facility (ALF) management staff.
  - If there is a living will; what is designated?
  - Original document location and who has access?
  - Where are copies located?
- Are there any religious practices that need to address?
  - Clergy contact information
  - Is clergy aware?
  - Who will contact the clergy?

Note: some states have additional physician pre-signed DNR/DNAR paperwork to be kept at home if EMS responds in an emergency. Having this paperwork available will ensure that EMS will abide by your loved one's wishes. Keep documents on the refrigerator and/or by the bedside.

Where Can Hospice Provide Services

Deciding where to receive hospice can be a very personal choice. Mom was adamant that she wanted to remain in her home. Hospice services can be provided in the home, independent living facility, ALF, Long Term Care (LTC)/nursing homes, and at inpatient hospice units. Short-term inpatient hospice services may be provided in a hospital or free-standing hospice facility.

Some hospice services are provided by home health agencies that coordinate services at the residence, ALF, or nursing home. The agency may contract for an inpatient hospice bed should extensive symptom management be needed. There are also hospice entity programs offering comprehensive hospice services no matter where your loved one is living and have their own inpatient facilities. Learn about available hospice services in your community, and speak with medical professionals, including physicians, case managers, and social workers, to help you in the decision-making process.

Your loved one may transition from an independent living setting to one requiring additional assistance and care, or intensified services may be offered to keep them living in-place. When a living location is changed, the hospice paperwork must be reviewed and, in some cases, resigned. It is similar to the initial lengthy admissions process. The process is designed to ensure that all aspects of care are reviewed and that the transition to the new setting takes place safely.

When Hospice Discontinues Benefits

With good care and symptom management, individuals may go in to remission, stabilize, even improve for a while, and hospice care may no longer be needed. Should this happen and hospice criteria are no longer met, you will be responsible for obtaining and coordinating the needed continuing care. When hospice discontinues benefits it means that your loved one will no longer have the previously provided hospice personal care, nursing, medical equipment (hospital bed, over-bed table, oxygen, lifts, wheelchair, etc.) and other support services. Hospice should provide several days of notice to the loved one or the healthcare proxy; this should not be a surprise. You will need to quickly identify and secure new personal care providers to minimize a gap in care for your loved one.

The discontinuation of hospice services means that there may now be additional bills since medications and supplies related to the hospice diagnosis are no longer covered by hospice. There also may be additional expenses relating to personal care services for which the individual has a deductible or coinsurance payment. Coordination with hospice and the primary care or treating physician is necessary to clarify what continuing care is needed; services and equipment must be in place when hospice stops providing care. Ideally, the hospice staff should communicate with the new home care agency that will provide care, to minimize care issues. This hand-off communication will help ensure that that care continues seamlessly.

Revoking Hospice Benefits

Hospice care can be revoked at any time by the hospice recipient. Some of the reasons for disenrolling can include: pursue treatments not covered under hospice (radiation, chemotherapy, clinical trial, experimental), or moving to an area where there is no hospice. Should the decision be made to revoke hospice care, a revocation form must be signed, indicating, the date hospice care will end. A revocation cannot be done verbally. Be sure to ask about any exclusion period and how it may impact your loved one.

Non-Medicare & Medicaid beneficiaries should contact their insurance company to determine the process and associated implications of disenrollment and reenrolling. Be sure to consult with hospice on your specific circumstances and address any concerns upfront before revoking the benefit.

Discharge for Cause

There may be extraordinary circumstances in which a hospice is unable to continue providing hospice care to an individual.

- When a hospice determines that the individual's (or other persons in the home) behavior is disruptive, abusive, or uncooperative so that the delivery of care or the ability of the hospice to operate effectively is seriously impaired, the hospice can consider discharge for cause

- The hospice must make every effort to resolve these problems before it can consider discharge for cause as an option. The hospice may also need to make referrals to other relevant agencies as appropriate

- The hospice must do the following before it discharges an individual for cause:
  - Advise the individual that a discharge for cause is being considered

- o Make a serious effort to resolve the problem(s) presented by the individual's behavior or situation

The Four Levels of Hospice Care

There are four levels of hospice care services. There may be a progression in services based on individual needs, preferences or medical status.

- **Routine home care**—available wherever your loved one considers home (private residence, nursing home, assisted living community). The hospice team members visit your loved one, usually singly and at varying intervals based on a routine that is determined by the plan of care. This could be daily, semiweekly, or weekly depending on your loved one's needs.
- **Continuous Care**— Intensive Symptom Management/provided in the home in continuous shifts of up to 24 hours by hospice nurses and aides during brief periods of crisis. As an example, this level of care would be appropriate if your loved one's medical needs required constant monitoring in the home, nursing home or assisted living community.
- **Inpatient hospice care**—provided in an inpatient hospice unit or bed in a designated healthcare facility for a short period when your loved one's medical needs cannot be managed at home.
- **Respite care**—the individual being cared for at home is offered a short stay in an inpatient setting to give family members and other caregivers a rest, or when they need to be away.

Considerations:

- What does your loved one want?
- Where is the best place for care?
- Can the location accommodate the equipment, caregivers, and family?
- If hospice care is provided at home, who will be the primary caregiver?
- If around the clock care is needed, who will provide it?

- Who can be part of the caregiving circle?
- If the needs change, can the care be adjusted or provided in a different location?

The Hospice Team

Many hospice professionals are available to assist your loved one and family. It is important to remember hospice services vary between hospices, and that some services may not be needed or desired. The focus of the hospice team is to keep your loved one comfortable, addressing pain and symptom management, including muscle stiffness, swallowing difficulties, breathing, hydration, nutrition, infections, anxiety, depression, communication, and other individual concerns. Hospice team members that are frequently encountered include:

- **Hospice physician** is specially trained in the care and comfort of dying individuals participates in the development of the plan of care, consults on comfort measures, and works together with the personal physician when requested
- **Advanced Practice Registered Nurse** (ARNP), also known as Advanced Practice Nurse or Nurse Practitioner, is a registered nurse who completes a graduate-level program and has additional clinical education, skills and responsibilities for administering patient care. Depending on the state, they may have prescribing authority and can practice independently and often work as physician extenders
- **Registered Nurse** (RN) regularly visits to monitor the medical condition, provides care and comfort, coordinates medications and medical equipment orders, and reports condition updates to the hospice physician and personal physician
- **Social Worker** (SW) provides emotional support and helps the family access financial and community resources, and end-of-life planning
- **Certified Nursing Assistant** (CNA) helps with personal care and hygiene, light housekeeping, light laundry, and occasional shopping and meal preparation

- **Chaplain** offers spiritual and emotional support and can work with your clergy
- **Community volunteer** offers companionship and respite relief
- **Bereavement specialist** offers support and groups for loved ones

Other specialists such as dietician or wound care nurse may be brought in to address or consult on specific issues. Their recommendations are then incorporated into the Plan of Care.

Hospice team member's roles and responsibilities.

The Hospice Team members are there to support your loved one and the family. Collectively, the individuals supporting the person in hospice are known as the Circle of Care, and their roles are well-defined. The diagram shows the core members and key roles, and responsibilities for that position. Depending on the hospice you select there may be some additional support team members.

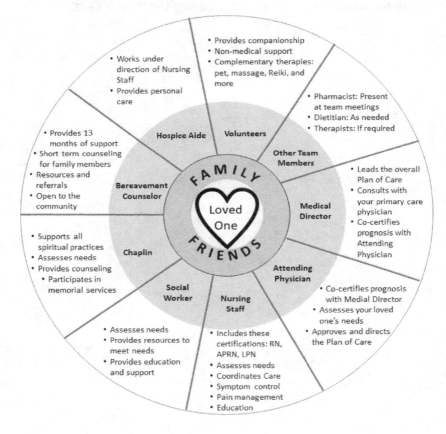

 Issues for discussion when initiating hospice care:

- What are our care wishes?
- What care do we think is needed?

- What are the specific medical issues and symptoms to be managed?
- What non-medical issues need to be addressed (bill paying, food shopping, laundry, etc.)?
- What resources do we have to assist (financial, equipment, support, etc.)?
- Which hospice professionals and services are needed?
- Does the hospice we are considering have the specially trained staff who can meet our needs?
- Are there spiritual or religious practices that need to be accommodated?
- Is your loved one and the family in agreement with the hospice approach and treatment plan, or is the assistance of a professional needed to bring clarity?
- Can the nurse, social worker, and clergy all come at one time for a joint (combined) appointment?
- When regularly assigned team members are not available and substitute caregivers are being made; be sure to ask about the timing of the visit. Often the substitute is asked to fit in the visit, and they may not arrive when usually expected.
- How is the information regarding your loved one and family preferences communicated to new team members? Often it is the family or caregivers who spend a lot of time sharing and re-sharing information with new hospice staff members.

Caregiving

The Circle of Care has a core group of professionals that you will most frequently interact with on a daily or weekly basis. These individuals will also facilitate the interaction with other professionals in the Circle of Care.

Physician

When a hospice is selected, an attending/primary physician is also chosen. The attending physician is responsible for the primary care of your loved one. This may be their long-standing physician or a hospice physician. Many people who receive hospice care at home remain with their physician, providing the physician is willing and able to coordinate care with the hospice.

There may be situations where physician care/treatment for your loved one may have additional financial implications. The differentiator is going to be whether the care/treatment is associated with the hospice diagnosis. Comfort care related to the hospice admitting diagnosis is usually reimbursed by hospice. When a physician treats your loved one for something not related to the hospice diagnosis you are responsible for the cost of care. As an example, an ophthalmologist is treating your loved one for ongoing glaucoma. This condition is not related to the hospice diagnosis, and the associated costs are not covered by hospice. If your loved one requires care from a practitioner other than the hospice physician, be sure to ask if hospice covers the physician fees. These situations tend to surface more frequently when loved ones are in hospice for a longer period of time.

Should you have questions or concerns, speak to the financial/billing staff at the hospice's administrative office. The nurses may not be up-to-date on all the financial implications of hospice billing. These billing rules are complex and are payor specific; it is best to clarify with knowledgeable individuals before incurring the bills.

Nursing

It takes a unique person to be a hospice nurse. They are your advocate. You may also see them as compassionate, empathetic, and caring individuals that you can lean on. A hospice nurse typically covers 16-20 hospice patients. The home visits normally take place weekly (there are some hospices where the nurse only visits every two weeks); depending on symptoms and clinical needs, visits **may** occur more frequently. Hospice nursing care is NOT intended to be "around-the-clock" and is not a substitute for other forms of caregiving. You can also expect to see a hospice nurse when there is a significant change in your loved one's condition when new or uncontrolled symptoms surface. During the visit, vital signs and symptoms will be assessed, medications reviewed, supplies inventoried, and a review of your loved one's and caregivers' status and issues will be addressed.

Certified Nursing Assistant (CNA)

A CNA is a very special person. They are they face your loved one will most frequently see. Their presence and attitude can help set the tone for the day. Over time, they may become the arms, legs, and eyes for your loved one. Eventually, they may even learn your loved one's nuances as well as you do. Your loved one and you need to feel comfortable with the CNA. There is a level of match-making that goes into finding the right CNA. Do not hesitate to speak with your nurse or scheduling department to help find a better CNA match.

The hospice CNA may have a daily caseload of up to 12 individuals. They work under the direct supervision of the RN and must adhere to the care plan established by the RN, based on the clinical status and needs. Please be aware; the CNA has restrictions on what activities can and cannot be performed. The CNA is in jeopardy when you ask them to perform a prohibited task. For example, a CNA is prohibited from opening or dispensing medication, even over-the-counter medicine.

The CNA typically is the individual that spends the most time with your loved one and reports any clinical changes to the RN for further assessment. The CNA's role revolves around addressing and assisting with the activities of daily living (ADL). ADLs include eating, bathing, toileting, dressing, management of incontinence, and transferring in and out of bed.

Personal Note: CNA coverage for many families is the challenge, and we were no exception. The hospice or home care agencies rarely have a substitute caregiver that can come at the pre-arranged time, should there be a last-minute call that the CNA will not be coming for the scheduled visit. Mom's CNA was the individual who got her up and out of bed three days a week. I was fortunate that mom could alert me when the CNA did not arrive as scheduled. Many times, I could get an alternate caregiver to her apartment, other times, I had to make an emergency run to get mom out of bed, fed, and medicated until the next caregiver came for the routinely scheduled visits.

Caregivers

Depending on your loved one's overall medical status when beginning hospice services, a family member or friend may already be serving in the caregiver role. Caregiving needs increase as the medical condition declines. There are three very important questions to ask:

1. Is the caregiver **able**? The caregiver may be willing and available, yet due to their age and own medical condition, are not be able to provide all needed care? Consider the physical size of your loved one and the caregiver (e.g., a 6', 225 lb. husband being managed by a 5', 90 lb. spouse with a heart condition). What is the extent and frequency of care needs, incontinence care, and repositioning every two hours? Is this individual physically able to meet the needs?

2. Is the caregiver **willing**? Does the caregiver truly want to be the individual providing the care? Is this person comfortable doing so? Balance this with the changing care needs. Is the caregiver emotionally capable of fulfilling your loved one's wishes (i.e., DNR)?

3.   Is there an **available** caregiver? Can the caregiver be there for all the needs? Does this person work, or have other responsibilities that will make them unavailable? Balance this with the changing care needs is very important.

Answering these questions at the onset of care and periodically during the hospice journey, will help determine if the caregiving arrangement are still appropriate, and may signal caregiver "burnout." Caregiving is stressful; it is an additional set of activities performed beyond one's daily routine. Care needs often become more complex and may be beyond the abilities of the caregiver. Caregiving may be shared between hospice staff and a caregiving circle, the patchwork of family, friends, and volunteers.

When caregiving needs are beyond what hospice, or the caregiving circle can provide, it is time to consider additional paid help.

 Consider:

- Are all caregivers dependable?
  - o Will they show up?
  - o Will they stay for the agreed upon timeframe?
  - o Is there a backup caregiver?
- Are special arrangements or accommodations needed for the caregivers?
  - o Do they need written instructions?
  - o Are they able to reach items needed for caregiving?
  - o Do containers or bottles need to be opened for them?
- Are caregivers able to follow the Plan of Care?
  - o Withhold (not-give) food or medication that the individual is not allowed to have?
  - o Would they withhold any medication, treatment, or assistance (walking or turning) that your loved one should have?

- Will the caregiver share any issues, concerns or problems with the designated contact person or the rest of the team?
- Is the caregiver able to emotionally handle the changes in the medical condition?
- How will you handle a cancellation or unavailability of a caregiver? Backup plans are vital!
- Who from the family is the main contact person?
- Who from the family is responsible for coordinating care?

Emergency contacts with phone numbers should be posted on the refrigerator, along with the medication sheet and DNR paperwork.

Paid Caregivers

Professional caregivers are often employed to assist with the routine, more strenuous and personal aspects of care (moving, toileting, and washing). Hospice may provide a CNA two or three times a week for up to one hour per visit, yet this may not be sufficient to meet the growing care needs of your loved one. When faced with the decision to hire help, it is important to find the right person, who can perform the care safely, with compassion, and is reliable. During mom's hospice stay, the paid CNA was invaluable to us. We thought of them as family, and they helped us through the tough times. Our lives were made better because of their care and support.

The consistency of caregivers is important, it builds trust, confidences and minimizes issues and errors in the care delivery process. Some families elect to find this person on their own, not taking into consideration the need for backup care, should the person call out (not show up for work), unable to perform required functions or may be untrustworthy. When using an agency, there are situations when caregivers are unavailable, and a substitute is being used to fill in; be sure to confirm the time of the visit. The visit to your loved one may be an additional task in their schedule, and may not be in keeping with the previous caregiver's schedule.

Financial factors that also need to be addressed when hiring help without going through an agency, including the tax implications of directly hired help. If you elect to pay a caregiver "under the table," without filing any tax or Social Security forms, you expose yourself to possible penalties and fines by the IRS. Working with a licensed and bonded agency that performs a background check, offers worker's compensation, and monitors the care provided helps to alleviate these issues. No matter which agency you select, ask and investigate the background of the owners, and be sure that you know who is supervising the caregivers. Websites like Medicare.gov Home Health Compare ✎, Center for Medicare & Medicaid Services (Home Health Star Ratings) ✎, and Department of Health and Human Services (Eldercare Locator) ✎ may help provide you insights into some agencies. The issue of caregiver dependability and consistency is one of the most frequently shared frustrations by families. There are times that the agencies do not have "replacement" staff available to keep the caregiving appointment. It is critical that you have back–up care arrangements. It is especially important when bad weather is expected (snow storms and hurricanes), and roads may not be drivable.

Caregiver registries can help you locate an independent caregiver. You will negotiate directly with that individual, and you can decide when to make a caregiving change. The Caregiver Registry can be a backup resource should the agency be unable to staff and you have advance notice. It is important for you to determine if the caregiver is a right fit for your loved one. Meet with them on neutral ground (over coffee) and "listen" to your gut. Verify and validate all credentials and be sure to perform a background check (criminal, civil, abuse, and motor vehicles). When hiring from an agency these background checks have typically been performed. A list of registries that have been accredited by the Caregiver Registry Standards Board (CRSB) can be found online. ✎ It has a state by state listing of accredited registries. Some states require licensing for independent contractors. You can find them at Private Care Association. ✆

Cost of care depends on the geographical location where care is provided, and the amount of care needed. Extensive home care services are expensive and may easily amount to more than assisted living or nursing home placement. It is common to pay at least $20 per hour, with a minimum booking of four, six or eight-hour blocks of time. In some locations, the cost may be closer to $30 per hour. Some agencies may charge a premium for nights, weekends and holidays. A quick cost calculation: at $20 per hour, one day of care (24 hours) costs $480; for 30-days, that cost would be $14,400 excluding any premium charges. It is very important to be aware of hired care costs since they add up quickly and can place the individual and family in a financial bind.

If your loved one is residing in an independent living facility, they may have access to "shared care." Shared care is an emerging concept where several residents "share" a caregiver who assists with bathing, toileting, dressing, meal preparation, and medication reminders. A shared caregiver may make several scheduled visits during the day. These individuals do not need constant care, and the periodic care has been evaluated to meet needs and considers safety factors. Cost of this care has a slightly higher hourly cost, yet there may not be a minimum booking of hours. Often an individual may be able to start with such an arrangement and then increase services as needed.

If Long Term Care (LTC) Insurance was purchased, this is an ideal time to activate it. Depending on the policy, being enrolled in hospice may defer the Functional Assessment and the Elimination Period. Contact the LTC insurance carrier as soon as possible; they often can provide the names of caregiving agencies in your area to assist. It is important to know what the LTC policy actually covers. Early policies written in the 1980 and 1990 may only cover $100-$150 per day of care. Policies written more recently may be for a specified total dollar amount available for care. If care needs are not extensive and the policy's total daily benefit allowance is not used, (e.g., using $100 of a $120 per day policy) the unused funds are lost and not available for future use.

How would you handle it ... call out of the caregiver

"I'm Joan from the hospice scheduling department. I wanted to let you know that Keisha, your CNA, will not be there tomorrow at 7 AM. Shirley will be there at 10 AM instead." Mom is 94, and dependent on others to walk with her since she is at risk for falls. For the last two months, Keisha has been getting mom out of bed on Mondays, Wednesdays, and Fridays, reminding her to take her meds, walking her to the bathroom, giving her breakfast and placing her in a chair. The other caregivers' schedule is based on when the hospice CNA makes her visits. Joan's last-minute call results in a frantic series of phone calls to the home care agency to alter the schedule of the other caregivers. You have just been told that the home care staff cannot modify their schedule on such short notice. Mom needs to be cared for now. A few important immediate needs that can't be delayed include toileting, medications, and breakfast.

A call out is a common type of call. It means the regular CNA will not be coming that day. In this example, at least there was some advanced warning. You should anticipate such an occurrence on weekends, holidays. When a staff member calls out, how will you handle such a situation?

- Which member of the circle-of-care can get to mom the quickest? Failure to have mom cared for may result in an injury or viewed as neglect.
- Do you have a list of backup agencies for caregiving assistance?
- Has mom been told of the change to her routine and advised of how her needs will be met?

A list of Medicare certified agencies in your area can be found online at the Medicare.gov website. ✎ The website provides general agency information, Quality of Care ratings, and Patient Survey results. Information on staff reliability or communication skills is not provided, yet the information is helpful in narrowing down agency choices. It is always good to get recommendations from family, friends, and healthcare professionals on their experiences with various agencies.

Medicare has published a Home Health Agency checklist to assist you in selecting an agency. ✎

Practical Caregiving

If there is one word I would ask you to embrace as you embark on this hospice journey, it would be "patience." You may learn amazingly positive things about yourself, the circle of care, and people outside the circle. You may also learn about their limits. As you do learn, be patient. Everyone handles stress and loss differently.

It is very important that your loved one and family members take the time to understand what they expect of each other and the professionals involved in medical management and caregiving. Don't assume anything. Identify the tasks and responsibilities that each individual involved in caregiving will take on. Leave nothing to chance! The more that is discussed and agreed upon up front, the more it will help mitigate surprises and disappointments. Remember, some individuals are better suited for direct caregiving than others, yet everyone can do something to relieve the stress of caregiving. Many families find a written calendar or guide to be very helpful.

 Consider defining responsibilities for:

- Meal preparation
- Medication management (filling pill boxes, giving medications, refilling prescriptions and remaining up-to-date on all medications being given)
- Ordering supplies
- Washing and toileting
- Doing the laundry
- Housecleaning
- Paying bills
- Food shopping
- Caring for pets
- Running errands

What can your loved one do safely independently? Their independence level will change over time. Be sure that expectations are re-evaluated as conditions change.

- Can caregivers turn, lift, move, bath, feed and transport your loved one safely?
- Can your loved one be left alone for the caregiver to go shopping?
- Calling hospice when there's a change in condition or an emergency:
    - Who in the circle of care should be contacted next?
    - Has a call tree or email contact group been established? Relieve one person from having to contact everyone by phone to share the communication.
- Can medication be managed safely? Is dosing complicated and variable?

No question is too small or silly. A concern of yours must be addressed, and the worry factor removed.

Situation: the caregiver spokesperson

Harry, a widower, is no longer able to manage his affairs (pay bills, food shop, keep track of his medications, at times forgetful) and has asked his daughter Jane to step in. Harry has an Advance Directive naming his daughter Jane who lives several miles away to serve on his behalf. Harry's son, Tom is older than Jane; he lives out of state, frequently travels and has not been keeping in touch with Harry and Jane. Tom has been calling the hospice physician, nurse, and social worker; additionally, he will not speak with his sister. Tom has also arranged to have food brought in for his father, yet the items he selects are made in heavy sauces and are too tough for Harry to chew. Harry's third child Margaret has been close to her father, also lives out of the area and is very concerned about her father's status and has also been calling members of the hospice team. She has been sending some supplies not covered by hospice.

- Jane and Harry must speak with Tom and Margaret to share why the hospice wants to communicate with one family spokesperson (it avoids conflicting directives, and there are legal issues). There may be exceptions to this practice and a weekly conference call with hospice may be a solution so that everyone in the family hears the updates at the same time.
- Have the hospice dietician communicate with Tom the types of foods that Harry can eat and share that with the individuals preparing the meals.

Clean, Clean, Clean

Handwashing is very important in keeping your loved one from getting an infection and keeping caregivers free from illness. Handwashing should be done before and after direct contact or care for your loved one. Wearing of gloves does not eliminate the need for handwashing. All visitors should be asked to wash their hands before coming in contact with your loved one.

When should you wash your hands

Feces (poop) from people or animals, is an abundant source of germs. A single gram of human feces, which is about the weight of a paper clip, can contain one trillion germs. Help stop the spread of germs by washing your hands often, especially during these key times:

- **Before**, during, and after preparing food
- **Before** eating food
- **Before** and after caring for someone who is sick
- **Before** and after treating a cut or wound
- **After** using the toilet
- **After** changing a diaper or use of the toilet
- **After** blowing your nose, coughing, or sneezing
- **After** touching an animal, animal feed, or animal waste
- **After** touching garbage

What is the right way to wash your hands? Follow these five steps to wash your hands the right way every time:

- **Wet** your hands with clean, running water (warm or cold), and apply soap.
- **Lather** your hands by rubbing them together with the soap. Be sure to lather the backs of your hands, between your fingers, and under your nails.
- **Scrub** your hands for at least 20 seconds. Need a timer? Hum the "Happy Birthday" song from beginning to end twice.
- **Rinse** your hands well under clean, running water.
- **Dry** your hands using a paper towel or a clean towel.

What about hand sanitizers? A hand sanitizer is not a substitute for washing your hands. It won't clean visibly dirty hands and is not as effective as soap and water in killing most germs.

How to use hand sanitizers:

- **Apply** the product to the palm of one hand (read the label to learn the correct amount).
- **Rub** your hands together.
- **Rub** the product over all surfaces of your hands and fingers until your hands are dry.

The CDC's guidelines on handwashing can be found on their website. ✎

When soap and water are not available, use an alcohol-based hand sanitizer that contains at least 60% alcohol. **If your loved one has C-difficile or norovirus (causes stomach pain, nausea, diarrhea, and vomiting), then handwashing is a must, and hand sanitizers should <u>NOT</u> be used**.

Home Safety Considerations

A major challenge in providing care is to ensure that the environment is safe for everyone. Depending on the condition, strength, alertness, and mobility level some home modifications may be needed. Key issues to address include: clutter, items on the floor that could be a trip hazard, lighting, ability to safely shower and toilet, and securing of medication. Preventing falls is a very important part of the home safety evaluation. Should your loved one have decreased mental functioning and wander, then additional measures will be required to ensure a safe environment. As their status changes, additional safety considerations may be needed. Be sure to discuss these specific issues with your hospice nurse.

 For home care, consider if the home can accommodate the equipment and staff needs, given home size, location, power needs, and available financial and physical resources. Items to take into account around the home include:

- Appropriate lighting; night lights available for the bathroom, bedroom & kitchen
- Flooring intact (no carpet buckling, loose floor tiles or trip hazards)
- Appropriate temperature control
- Grab bars in the bathroom for the shower and near the toilet, or 3:1 commode that goes over the toilet and can also be placed in the shower
- Non-slip shower or tub surface
- Phone, TV, and lighting control is near the bed
- Ability to secure medications. This is important if the individual wanders or has confusion. Narcotics should be secured and not left out in the open.
- Trip or slip hazards (scatter rugs, power cords across floor, furniture or equipment)
  - Does anything need to be rearranged to ensure a more direct path between rooms?
  - Are gates needed at the top or bottom of staircases?
- Doorframes sufficiently wide and room configuration; accommodating medical equipment including wheelchair or raised commode
- Items within easy reach, minimizing the need to bend or stretch
- Handrails for stairs

- Carpet on stairs secured
- Smoke detector
- Fire extinguisher
- Review the outside entrances to the residence, checking for trip hazards, loose hand railings, lighting

You have to assess what your loved one can do safely independently, and this will change over time. Be prepared for changing needs. If dementia or altered mental status is an issue, then additional factors need to be considered:

- Securing or removing range and oven controls
- Installing light sensors
- Install technology that will alert when doors or windows are opened
- Hiding a key where your loved one cannot access it

Two good reference documents are:

The Consumer Product Safety Commission's Safety for Older Consumers-Home Safety Checklist ✎

CDC Check for Safety – A Home Fall Prevention Checklist for Older Adults ✎

Hospice Medication Pack - Comfort/Emergency Medications

Once your loved one is signed-up for hospice services, a special medication box will be delivered to the home. This box of comfort/emergency medications should be stored in the refrigerator. The medications in the box are to be used only at the direction of hospice staff to alleviate a variety of distressing symptoms (pain, nausea, constipation, difficulty breathing, anxiety, and insomnia). In some instances, the box may be customized to the diagnosis or unique needs. *It is important that the box is kept secured and not opened until directed to do so by the hospice clinical staff*. Having these medications handy, and used according to directions, means that various distressing symptoms can be addressed quickly. Unfortunately, there are caregivers and others who are dependent on narcotics; and this type of medication also has a high "street value." Some of the medications in the box may be narcotics, and the contents of the box need to be regularly inventoried to ensure that the medications are accounted for.

Medications

Medication Management is one of the most critical aspects of caregiving. The correct administration (giving) of medications is critical to condition and symptom management. Medication administration becomes harder when there are several caregivers assisting the individual with taking medications. Record all medications given on a Medication Administration Record (MAR). A sample form is available in the Resource section (Medication Administration Record, Appendix A.) and on www.JudithSands.com. It is helpful to have the routine prescription medications listed on the top of the form, and those used for symptom management at the bottom of the page. Be sure to include as-needed over the counter items like vitamins, nutritional supplements, stool softeners, enemas, and pain analgesics. Hospice will provide or cover medications that are **directly related to the reason for admission**. For example, pain medication for a diagnosis of cancer will be covered, yet the blood pressure pills would not be covered because blood pressure management was not the reason for the hospice services. Also, a co-payment may be required. Over-the-counter medications are not typically covered. Be sure to discuss specific medication issues with the hospice nurse. **If Medicare Part D coverage has been purchased, do not automatically discontinue it. Medicare Part D coverage may be very helpful, especially if hospice is not covering all of the routine medications needed for care**.

There is a big variation in the cost of medications not covered by hospice, even with insurance. Be sure to compare prices between pharmacies, big box stores, and shopping clubs. You will be amazed at what you can save. Often transferring a prescription can result in a gift card of about $25. It is important to keep medications with the same pharmacy to minimize any medication interactions.

Often pain management is a primary goal for the hospice team. Typically, there is a progression from over-the-counter to prescription medications. Narcotics are often prescribed to manage and relieve the symptoms. There are times that other types of therapy may be used to relieve pain. One of the most common side effects of narcotics is constipation (hard stools), and it is important to use stool softeners, including products containing psyllium that may be used on a daily basis. Eating fiber-rich foods such as prunes, apricots, and figs, along with sufficient fluid intake is also very important. Mobility is also an essential consideration; whenever possible encourage the most activity that can be tolerated safely. Depending on the type, number, and quantity of narcotics being given, the level of alertness and wakefulness will begin to be impacted and increased periods of sleepiness will be seen.

Narcotic (pain management) medications is a category of medications that are often abused in the general population. To minimize the possibility that the narcotic medications will be taken or stolen, **do not leave them in plain sight.** Having these medications out of sight will help ensure that the medication is always available for the individual.

 Consider:

- Keep a list of all medications (prescribed & un-prescribed, vitamins, and supplements), dosages and times given
- Take a copy of the medication list, including updates to each physician visit
- Provide a copy of the continually updated medication list to the caregiver and designated family member(s)
- Routine pain medication schedule set up with hospice staff to keep pain manageable. Determine what medication will be used for "breakthrough pain"; the pain that is severe and it is not yet

time to take the next regularly scheduled dose of pain medication
- Repositioning to minimize stiffness and discomfort
- Make a homemade heating pad by pouring uncooked rice into a cotton sock and tie it off; heat the sock in the microwave for 1 minute, wrap in a thin towel and use it for localized pain or stiffness. Only use it if your loved one can tell if it is too hot, as the skin may be sensitive. DO NOT use heating pads.
- Use of stool softeners, psyllium, prunes and high fiber foods regularly to prevent constipation
- Keeping a chart (marking a calendar) when there is a bowel movement. This is very important especially when there are multiple caregivers, and the information may not be passed along
- Evaluate the drugs being covered by hospice against all medications needed to determine if Medicare Part D coverage should be continued. Ask your hospice nurse or pharmacist for assistance in reviewing your specific situation
- Narcotic medications need to be secured and not left out in plain view
- The hospice comfort medication pack should be refrigerated. This contains several medications that should only be used when instructed by the hospice nurse or doctor

When to Call the Hospice Nurse

New symptoms and unmanaged symptoms should be reported to the hospice nurse or on-call staff once recognized, do not delay in sharing condition changes. The staff is available to assist you by phone or will schedule a nurse to visit, as indicated by the severity of the symptom. The nurse should be called when there is:

- Ineffective pain management
- Difficulty or change in breathing or shortness of breath, congestion
- No bowel movement in 3 days

- Ongoing diarrhea
- Change in balance, coordination or strength
- Change in mental status (level of consciousness, responsiveness, awareness, confusion) or behavior
- New dizziness or fever
- Restlessness or agitation
- Decrease in the amount of urine
- New coolness of the hands, arms, feet, or legs

Nutrition

Adequate food intake is very important for comfort and quality of life. Work with your hospice team on finding foods that will minimize symptoms and constipation. Often frequent small snacks, finger foods are best tolerated. Modifications may need to be made when there are chewing or swallowing difficulties. As activity level decreases so does appetite. Sometimes the best way to encourage intake is to offer familiar favorite foods in small portions. Ethnic or regional foods may be a comfort, yet a challenge to caregivers who may be unfamiliar with the item and depending on the food item to be unappealing or unappetizing. Be prepared to educate the caregivers and share information about the various food items.

At the end-of-life, there is a natural, gradual decrease in thirst and hunger. In many cultures and families, food is a central part of life. It can be very distressing to family members and caregivers when an individual loses their appetite and interest in food.

 Consider:

- Safety with eating. What modifications need to be made to food preparation? Chopping or blending, thickening fluids to prevent choking, decreasing salt or sugar use, smaller portions and more frequent meals
- Addition of fiber and fluids to minimize constipation

- Some individuals will prefer their food to be less spicy while others will be seeking more flavorful foods
- Foods with a strong odor may no longer be appealing
- Provide small portions of food, pre-cut and ready for snacking
- Label and date food (including a discard date). This makes it easy for the caregiver to locate and serves as a prompt for when food should be discarded. This is especially important if there are multiple caregivers

Personal Note: Caregivers can say the funniest things! A backup paid caregiver came to get mom up, and give her breakfast. Mom requested a sandwich for breakfast. The caregiver, not accustomed to mom's request for non-traditional breakfast food called her supervisor for permission to comply. The supervisor instructed her to "give mom whatever she wants, and if she asks for a glass of wine, give it to her." Mom got her sandwich and declined wine at breakfast.

Family Conflicts

End-of-life discussions may be a time when unresolved family issues raise their heads. Often this is seen when estranged siblings or children surface after a prolonged period of no contact, or they have adopted beliefs and values that are not in keeping with the loved one. These individuals may oppose the loved one's prearrangements and impose their approach for end-of-life management. It is important that the loved one's wishes are respected and honored. At times, legal intervention may be necessary. The use of clergy or another respected individual advocate may be needed. A physician may be called upon to provide information on the medical condition.

On-Call, After-hours, Weekend and Holiday

Hospice must have core key services available during non-routine business hours (evenings, nights, weekends, and holidays). Staffing on the off-hours involves an On-Call team that is responsible for handling a "crisis," such as changes in status, providing guidance, obtaining emergent orders from physicians, emergencies, and pronouncing at the time of death. These staff members are not the "replacement" for the regular staff, yet are available to assist with unusual and challenging issues that families encounter outside of routine business hours. The impact to you may be longer wait times, less support staff available, and more interaction with answering services. Be prepared to wait for callbacks, and the need to repeat your issues and concerns multiple times.

Financial Considerations

As their physical status declines, your loved one will not be able to manage their financial affairs. Financial, and potentially legal, arrangements need to be identified so that bills can be paid, care rendered, food and supplies obtained while protecting the financial assets.

 Consider:

- Who will pay bills?
- Who can legally write a check and pay bills?
- Do bank accounts include the designated individual as one able to access financial records?
    - Are there any pre-signed checks?
    - Has an individual been legally designated a surrogate?
    - Is legal intervention needed?
    - Has electronic access to financial accounts been set up?
- Who has access to a safe deposit box on behalf of the individual?
    - Is their name registered with the bank?
    - Do they know where the safe deposit key is located?
- Who will manage the process for paying State and Federal Taxes (quarterly and annual payments)?
- Has a Last Will & Testament been drawn up for the individual in the state where death is anticipated?

- Where is the Last Will & Testament? It should only be kept in a safe deposit box if the executor has legal access to the box prior death. Leaving it with an attorney or trusted friend is a good option. It is important to keep it in a safe place and that the executor and beneficiaries know where it is located.
- Have funeral arrangements been made? Costs can be surprising, starting at $7,000-$10,000. Costs may be higher in some areas of the country, and there will be additional charges with placing the obituary in the newspaper and buying flowers. Cremation fees are noted to average $2,000-$4,000. As the size of the funeral grows, so do the expenses.
  - The Social Security survivors benefit program pays a special one-time lump sum amount (called the "Death Benefit") of $255 to help pay for funeral or burial costs for anyone who had qualified for Social Security benefits
  - To find out how to apply for this benefit, contact your local Social Security office or call 1-800-772-1213 (TTY 1-800-325-0778). Social Security Administration Web site page A Special Lump Sum Death Benefit ✏
  - Railroad Retirement and Survivor Benefits - there are benefits available to the surviving widow(er), children and other dependents. Contact: U.S. Railroad Retirement Board, 844 North Rush Street, Chicago IL, 60611-1275. Toll-Free: (877) 772-5772. TTY: (312) 751-4701. Directory: (312) 751-4300 ✏
  - US Department of Veterans Affairs – Burial Benefits. There are funds allocated for both Service-related and Non-service related deaths, and there are eligibility requirements. Contact the VA for further assistance and guidance ✏
  - Funeral Cost and Pricing Checklist from the Federal Trade Commission ✏

Funeral Pricing Checklist

Appendix C. is a checklist of items to consider when pricing a funeral. Use it to check with several funeral homes to compare costs.

Managing Expenses – Cost Savings

Medication and personal care items are costly. It is important to shop around and become knowledgeable of the cost of medications and supplies, especially if they are not related to the hospice diagnosis. Explore the prices of wholesale stores, big box stores, internet vendors and your local retailers. Some medical suppliers will work with individuals. Your hospice can help guide you in locating applicable resources.

Medical Equipment and Supplies

Medical equipment required for taking care of your loved one is typically provided by hospice; this includes a bed, specialty mattresses, over-bed table, commode or shower chair, a lift for getting out-of-bed, walker, wheelchair or other specialized items. The piece of equipment must be medically indicated to be covered by hospice.

Hospice will usually provide (this is also dependent on the type of medical insurance that you have) supplies that are needed for the care including: diapers, wipes, personal cleaning products, gloves, and dressing supplies. Note that not all hospices will provide the diapers, wipes, and cleaning products (this is also dependent on the type of medical insurance that you have). Be sure to ask up front what will be provided and how often supplies will be sent to the home. Check for any shipping or return fees. Some items you may be able to order in bulk while others should be ordered in smaller quantities given the individual's continuing need for the item. Many hospices deliver or ship supplies on a weekly schedule. There may be times that you will have to be the advocate and ask for additional or unanticipated supplies. It is not uncommon for hospice staff to drop off needed supplies on their way home.

Should the hospice not provide the diapers, wipes, and nutritional supplements, shop around for best pricing. Consider big-box stores, shopping clubs, and Internet stores as cost-cutting options.

Consider:

- It is important to know how to work each piece of equipment
  - Safety aspects such as always using the breaks on a wheelchair or rolling walker
  - Use side rails on the bed, when the individual is unsteady or wanders
  - Use of specialty mattress, foam, pillows or cushions to maintain a position and minimize pressure points
- Equipment and supply needs may change. Share concerns with the hospice staff, they can help make modifications to meet your loved one's needs
- Supply inventory levels are important; too much or too little supplies can challenge caregivers. Be sure to have an "emergency" stash of commonly used items (diapers, wipes, dressing supplies, etc.) so that you are not scrambling if the supplies did not arrive as planned. Supply levels will change as the individual's condition changes.
  - Track the number of diapers and dressing used per day to help with ordering
  - Ensure there are gloves for performing personal care
  - Reorder medications several days before the last dose is used

Utility Interruptions or Pending Adverse Weather Conditions

An interruption in electrical power can have a catastrophic impact on those dependent on electrical medical equipment. Beyond maintaining the comforts of heating and air conditioning, electricity is required for ventilators and oxygen compressors. Most electrical outages are for short periods of time; do not wait to call your oxygen vendor to advise them of the outage and need for backup oxygen. They need sufficient time to obtain and transport additional emergency oxygen. Pending adverse weather conditions (snow, hail, rainstorms, and hurricanes) are often known in advance. Oxygen and supply vendors usually have a plan to provide additional supplies in advance. Do not assume you have sufficient oxygen/supplies, contact your vendor or hospice staff directly as early as possible, to ensure that you will have the necessary items on hand before a change in weather conditions.

How would you handle ... the upcoming storm

You have just heard that the three-day weather forecast for your area includes a storm warning and winds are expected to be 40 MPH or greater. In the past, power outages and flooding are common. Your loved one requires an oxygen compressor to provide continuous oxygen. You have a portable tank that holds about 6 hours worth of oxygen. How will you handle such a situation?

- Check the fill level of the portable tank; fill the tank from the compressor
- Contact the oxygen vendor to request additional portable and large cylinders to ensure coverage during the storm
- Review with the oxygen vendor if local EMS is aware of oxygen dependence and their ability to provide backup

Loss of Independence

People enter hospice at different times based on their clinical condition. Those who are more alert, are stabilized and have their symptoms managed often are frustrated by their loss of body functions or independence. They may now be dependent on others for toileting which impacts their sense of dignity and self-image. Focus on those things that the individual may be able or can control. These could include the choice of what to wear, eat, watch or simple activities that they can perform. Provide choices that are in keeping with their condition. It is okay to ask if they would like to make the decision or would like it handled by someone else. Recognize that decision making abilities will decrease over time as their condition changes; being included in the decision-making process is often appreciated.

Health Information Portability & Accountability Act (HIPAA)

Your loved one will be asked to sign Notice of Privacy documents with each healthcare provider (hospice, physicians, durable medical equipment vendors). Be sure that these documents list the Healthcare Surrogate and any individuals that your loved one wishes to have access to their medical information. Do not rely on the Power of Attorney or Living Will forms. Access to these forms is often delayed.

Ask Me 3

When speaking with the hospice team, it is important to be sure that you and the individuals involved in caregiving understand instructions and ask for clarification. Asking questions helps ensure you have an understanding of what is occurring and helps provide caregivers with the rational and follow-through activities. The National Patient Safety Foundation (NPSF) suggested questions have been modified for the hospice setting:

- What is the main problem at this time?
- What needs to be done?
- Why is it important to do this?

Caregiver Communication

To ensure that the care focus remains on the needs of your loved one, a verbal "hand-off" between caregivers should take place with each change in caregivers. This communication between caregivers should be **clear**, **concise**, and **factual**. One approach is to review by topic:

Personal Care

- Issues with toileting, bathing, repositioning or turning; sharing any discomfort noted or shared, skin redness, bowel movements (constipation or diarrhea), and urination (issues with passing water)

- Issues with dressing, walking or movement

Medication

- Tolerance of routine medication
- Review the Medication Administration List (MAR)
  o Noting last doses of medications given
  o Need for pain or symptom management medications
- Breakthrough pain or uncontrolled symptoms

Food & Nutrition

- Amount and type of food and liquids taken
- Difficulty eating or swallowing
- Requests for special foods or foods to be limited

Any other issues

- Caregiver concerns
- Visitor encouragement or restriction
- Special requests

This handoff guide can also be found in Appendix E.

Consider:

- A notebook for caregivers with important contact information and key caregiving information
- A notebook page or form where all caregivers write issues, and there is a special section of items to discuss with the nurse and/or doctor
- Electronic tools or apps to assist in management are covered in a separate section

Visitors or No Visitors, That is the Question

When a care crisis surfaces, you will find that some friends will rally around you and others do not, due to their discomfort or insecurity about what to do, and they will be on the sidelines. Take advantage of those who offer to help and be specific in what you request of them. Individuals who are not comfortable with direct care may be delighted to shop or run errands for you. Don't overlook this type of help.

Deciding to encourage visitors is dependent on your loved one's status and wishes. Not everyone is at ease being seen when they are uncomfortable or surrounded by medical equipment. Reevaluate these visits based on your loved one's and caregiver status, and how the visitor behaves during the visit. You should not be entertaining these visitors; they should be providing emotional support, and at times, assistance. Have visitors call before they come and consider setting a 15-30 minute time limit on the visit based on how things are going. Do not be shy about telling visitors that they should come another time or need to leave so that caregiving or rest can take place.

Personal Note: Mom was known for her sayings. One of her favorites was: "Glad you could come, here's your hat, what's your hurry." The current version is better known as "don't let the door hit you on the ass on your way out."

Emotional and Caregiving Hospice Support

Clergy and social workers are skilled in helping with spiritual support and working through caregiving problems, including:

- Assisting in exploring non-medical ways to manage pain, anxiety, and symptoms
- Allow individuals and families to discuss their concerns and fears openly and without judgment
- Assist caregivers in finding support to maximize their strengths
- Assistance with insurance paperwork

- Identify community services and assist with setting up services, such as meals on wheels, lifeline, and others
- Provide caregivers with reading materials and information to support their role and to help them feel prepared for the time of death
- Help obtain financial assistance or resources
- Advocate for loved one's needs and concerns
- Assistance with funeral planning
- Assisting survivors with necessary arrangements and paperwork after death
- Assisting survivors in obtaining appropriate grief counseling

Caregiver Support

Caregivers are often stressed and tired from spending many hours providing care in addition to other responsibilities. When continuous caregiving and goes on for long periods of time, it may be necessary to ask for assistance. Many individuals do not like or feel comfortable asking for help.

Signs of caregiver stress
- Feeling exhausted all the time
- Getting sick more often than usual
- Not sleeping enough
- Feeling impatient, irritated, or forgetful
- Not enjoying things typically enjoyed
- Withdrawing from people

Common feelings expressed by caregivers
- Anxiety and worry – Worrying about how they will handle the additional responsibilities of caregiving and what will happen to your loved one if something happens to you. Fear of what will happen in the future as the illness progresses
- Anger or resentment – Resentfulness towards the person you're caring for, even though you know, it is irrational. Angry at the

world in general, or resentment of other friends or family members who don't have your responsibilities

- Guilt – Guilty for not doing more, being a "better" caregiver, having more patience, accepting of the situation, or in the case of long-distance caregiving, not being available more often
- Grief – Losses come with caregiving; the healthy future envisioned goals and dreams that will not be realized

Consider:

- Be specific when asking for help
    - "Please pick up the following items from the store for me"
    - "Please sit with my husband while I go to the pharmacy"
    - "Please replace a lightbulb in the ceiling for me"
    - "Please fix a meal for me once a week"
    - "Please walk the dog on Tuesdays"
- Locate a caregiver support group; often provided at hospices, churches, synagogues, and community centers
- Spend a few minutes each day focusing on what went well, and what you feel good about that happened during the day. Even in the face of illness and suffering, seek out the moments of joy and surprise. The individual's symptoms were better managed, they appeared comfortable, someone who unexpectedly provided support, the beauty of the day, the unanticipated greeting card
- Spend a few minutes journaling your feelings; use the power of the pen to share your private thoughts, and free your mind
- Do something just for yourself
    - Call a friend
    - Take a short walk, exercise, or nap
    - Take a hot bubble bath, have your hair or nails done

- Sit by yourself and enjoy a beverage for a few minutes
- Meditate, read a book, or pray
- Eat a nutritious meal
- Binge on chocolate or other treats

When caregivers are medical professionals

It is not uncommon for family caregivers with a medical background to become very involved with both the caregiving and the care coordination activities. These individuals often take on a major portion of the burden, especially if they are the spouse or children of the loved one. They often internally battle "intellect vs. emotions." These individuals need to be reminded of their familial roles and that it is okay not to be the "professional" always. "Cut yourself some slack!"

Acknowledge the Professional Caregivers

A little kindness goes a long way with the paid caregiver. Yes, you may be paying for their services, but it is not always easy or pleasant. Bringing a box of cookies or a meal for the team can be a simple way of showing them how much you appreciate their work. After all, they are taking care of your loved one, and you do want the best possible care. At the end of their service, a gratuity may be appropriate; check with the hospice that this does not violate policy. Let your heart help guide you on these matters.

Respite Care

Hospice can assist caregivers who need a temporary rest by moving your loved one to a nursing home, hospice inpatient facility or hospital. A hospice beneficiary can stay up to five days. Respite care can be utilized more than once, yet it only is provided on an occasional basis. There may be a need to pay 5% of the Medicare-approved amount for inpatient respite care. Speak to your hospice nurse to determine if you qualify for this occasional break in caregiving.

Unfinished Business

Many individuals have unfinished business! The business may be related to employment or professional responsibilities. For others it is very personal in nature; addressing friends and family with whom relationships have been great, or making a final peace or placing closure on a relationship that was broken in the past. Affording your loved one the option to address any unfinished business is a blessing to them, and to those around them. They may also need to hear from family and friends that they are valued and have "fought hard" and it is okay to pass on. Some individuals need that permission from their loved ones. Hearing is the last sense lost, so be sensitive as to what is said around your loved one. This is a great time to share final words of love and appreciation.

If your loved one utilizes hearing aids, be sure to replace the batteries often and clean the wax traps to ensure that your loving words are heard. If you are unable to clean the wax traps, takes the hearing aids to an audiologist or hearing aid vendor for service.

Consider:

- Is there someone that your loved one would like to speak with or have a letter sent expressing a particular message?
- Is there any work or other responsibilities that need to be delegated?
- Are there personal effects or items that they would like given away to a specific person or charity?
- Is there someone that should be notified of their condition so that they can reach out to them?
- Is there a desire for spiritual or religious support? Individuals may see comfort and support from clergy, even if they have not recently been actively involved with a religious community.

Saying Goodbye

Timeline for end-of-life changes:

Dying is a process. It involves the slowing of many bodily functions. Depending on the hospice diagnosis and progression of illness, the end-of-life process will be different for each individual. Focus on keeping your loved one comfortable, do not force food or drink, keep the environment calm, and free of loud noises and bright lights. Keep the skin clean, dry and moisturized, and protect from injury. Introduce yourself, although the individual may know you, they may not recognize you given their condition or because of being medicated. Position for comfort; this often involves keeping the head of the bed elevated to ease breathing. Medicate for symptom relief as directed by the hospice staff.

Personal Note: You may be faced with the situation as we were, that our hospice nurse was attending another family and the chain of symptom management became challenging. Although support was available by phone and guidance appreciated, a "crisis nurse" was sent. In our situation, this individual was not the model hospice nurse. She was not sensitive to the clinical information provided relating to the change in mom's comfort level, and the first words from her were "she looks comfortable to me." As previously noted, the last sense remaining is hearing. In the presence of mom, in a loud voice, she shared "your mother is now actively dying" and left. Within two minutes, mom became very agitated and aggressive comfort measures were needed, along with phone support from the hospice office. Hopefully, no one else will have to deal with a callous "professional," yet be prepared for the fact that valued support may be needed by phone.

One to Three Months

- Decreased desire for food
- Increased desire for sleep
- Withdrawal from people and the environment

Home Hospice Navigation

One to Two Weeks

- Sleep even more
- Confusion
- Restlessness
- Vision-like experiences
- Change in temperature, respiration, pulse, and blood pressure
- Congestion
- Not eating or a decreased intake of fluids
- Increased edema (swelling) of the arms, legs or body

Days or Hours

- Surge of energy
- Decreased blood pressure
- Glassy, teary eyes
- Half-opened eyes
- Irregular breathing
- Increased restlessness, confusion, disorientation
- Loss of consciousness
- Cold, purple, blotchy feet hands and earlobes
- Weak pulse
- Fever
- Decrease in amount of urine or very dark urine
- May say they are dying
- Loss of bowel and bladder control
- Talk about unfinished business

Minutes

- Gasping breathing or long pauses in breathing
- Inability to swallow
- No awakening
- Body held in rigid, unchanging position
- The jaw may drop or tilt to the side that the head is facing

Always remember that hearing may be last senses to go; be very sensitive as to what is said towards the end around the loved one. Be sure to express your love and share any last kind words for closure and peace at the time of death. **If your loved one utilizes hearing aids, be sure to replace the batteries often to ensure that your loving words are heard**.

End of Care/Time of Death

When the death happens, and no hospice staff member is with you, the first thing you need to do is call hospice and let them know that your loved one has died. Time of death will start a well-defined and scripted process; a chain of assistance will be provided to assist you. Hospice is the expert in managing all the activities once someone has died. A nurse (probably not your regular nurse) will come to the home to pronounce the passing. The nurse will assist you in contacting the funeral home, provide comfort, and the handle the removal of medical equipment, supplies, and hospice medications. The comfort pack may also be removed from the home. Not all hospice nurses are authorized to remove the comfort pack; be sure to ask for directions on how to properly dispose of the medications. **Narcotics used in keeping the individual comfortable will need to be destroyed to minimize the chance that they will be inappropriately used**.

Helpful Hints

Pill-Splitting

Pill-splitting may be needed when the medication is not available in the required dose. **It should only be done after checking with the ordering practitioner or pharmacist, as not all medications should be split**. Pill-splitting is a challenge when the tablet does not have a "score" (the manufactured indentation on some tablets shows the designated splitting point). A pill splitter can be purchased at your local pharmacy. It works best with scored pills. To split unscored pills, the easiest method I found, that does not leave tablet residue, involves a staple that has been stretched open and taped down with a piece of clear (cellophane) tape. Center the tablet over the taped down staple and lightly press down and the tablet will split into two pieces.

Chapped Lip Care

As the thirst desire lessens and there is less fluid intake, it is important to prevent lips from drying out and becoming chapped. There are many commercial lip care products available. Some contain petroleum jelly, and others contain beeswax, oils, and flavorings that may be unpleasant. A simple and cheap home remedy involves applying olive or vegetable oil to the lips with a cotton ball. Use a new cotton ball for each application.

Declutter

When caring for a loved one, your time and energies are shifted from your regular activities. Keeping the care area free of clutter, valuables, and breakables provides space for the caregiving equipment and lessens the change that valuables and breakables may be lost, misplaced, or broken. It also makes it easier to keep the area neat and clean. Caregivers often do not have the appreciation for your sentimental items. Removing valuables also reduces the temptation of less than honest caregivers for taking valuables. Theft is a real and unpleasant issue that some families confront. Do not be a victim! Increase your peace-of-mind by removing treasured items from view. Many families place jewelry in the bank vault or remove from the residence for safekeeping.

Barrier Cream

Skin is very sensitive and is easily irritated by moisture and bodily fluids (urine and feces). A specially formulated cream designed to keep moisture and bodily fluids (urine and feces) from irritating or relieving skin discomfort should be used with individuals who are not able to control their bladder or bowels. Barrier cream should be used on the skin after cleaning up from diarrhea.

Nausea (Queasy) & Vomiting

Your loved one may be nauseous continually or periodically. Nausea may be associated with headaches, bloating and cramps; causing physical and emotional distress. These symptoms may increase as death nears. Nausea and vomiting makes eating, drinking, and interacting with others very uncomfortable. Keep the room well ventilated and cool. Light, bland, dry carbohydrate (crackers, plain bread). Avoid fried and spicy foods, caffeine, smoking, sweets and sports drinks. Give small bland meals and have them eat slowly. Rest with the head elevated, especially after meals for at least 30 minutes. Wear loose-fitting clothes. Some medications can reduce nausea and vomiting; speak with your hospice nurse to identify the medication best suited for your loved one.

Odors & Smells

You and the caregiver need to be sensitive to the odors that arise from a variety of body fluids (urine, feces, vomit, sweat, and wounds), but also to the smells from cooking, smoking, perfumes, cleaning products and room deodorizers. Your loved one may find them to be bothersome and may complain of nausea. Fresh air is always a great option, yet may not be practical. Bodily fluids always need to be cleaned promptly, a few drops of mouthwash on a washcloth used during the bathing and toileting of your loved one may also decrease or eliminate body odor. Discuss any continuing smells with your hospice nurse. Ask visitors not to use perfume or body sprays before visiting, and avoid cooking or frying foods that may be offensive smelling. Consider putting a sign on the door to remind visitors about being perfume or cologne-free.

Pets

Dogs are known for sensing the onset of seizures and picking up the scent of some cancers; this may cause them to react differently to your loved one. Family pet's routine may be altered given a change in condition. Consider who will walk the dog, change the bird seed, and clean the rabbit droppings or litterbox. Depending on the type of animal and its needs, be sure that they are being met. This may be the time to ask a friend who is not comfortable with providing direct care to your loved one to assist in a different way.

Words of Comfort

Families and loved ones need emotional support during the dying process and after the individual has died. You will be amazed by who does, and who does not express condolences. A hug is wonderful, even if no words follow it. The emotions conveyed are powerful on their own. One most touching expression came from mom's letter carrier, a touching condolence note.

The following phrases represent general themes that convey caring; modify and expand as appropriate, sharing a touching memory:

- I am thinking of you
- I am a call away
- I am here for you
- I will do the following for you...
- I am here to help
- I am sorry you are suffering
- I am grateful to have known
- The "loved one" will be missed
- This is a tough time
- There are no words to
- May their memory be a blessing to you

- May good/happy memories help comfort you
- Remember the happy times shared
- Wishing you healing and comfort in memories
- Words are inadequate to express our sadness
- So sorry for your loss
- You are in my prayers
- My favorite memory of your loved one is ...

Handling Questions

Family and friends want to support you during this difficult time. Their discomfort with the situation may result in them inadvertently saying the wrong thing. It is not out of maliciousness, yet the words may come out as lacking consideration for the situation. It is important to remember that they want to comfort you and let you know how much they care. Do not to overreact. You may hear:

- I know how you feel
- How are you doing?
- You look terrible
- What's wrong with you?
- You are handling this better than I expected
- It could be worse
- No offense, but ...
- The "loved one" is in a better place
- Asking if estranged friends or family have been in touch, or attended the funeral
- Did the "loved one" suffer?
- Who did the "loved one" ask for?
- Well, what did the "loved one" die from?
- How did the "loved one" die?
- Did "the loved one" confess anything?
- Was dying like they show in the movies?
- You must be so relieved now that the "loved one" is gone
- Is there an inheritance?
- Can I have the "loved one's" belongings?

There is no right answer to these questions. Some of you will ignore the question; others may have a witty response, chastise the person for their callousness, or simply answer the question. A simple deflection response may be, such as "I appreciate your concern, but now is not a good time to discuss this." Remember, they may not have had the opportunity to read this book and understand everything you have experienced.

Comments/Corrections/Additions

Every effort has been made to provide a practical and useful resource to guide you through a very difficult and emotional time in your life. I may have missed an important topic for you, or your personal experience can enhance this book. I welcome your thoughts and look forward to hearing from you about your experiences.

Please consider leaving a brief book review on Amazon or Goodreads.

Thank you, Judith

Email: Judith@JudithSands.com

Website: www.JudithSands.com

Resources

There is an abundance of material on the topic of hospice, advanced care planning, and caregiving. Use reputable, professional sources when obtaining information from the Internet. The following resources are current as of this publication.

Websites

MedlinePlus is the National Institutes of Health's Web site for loved ones, their families, and friends. Produced by the National Library of Medicine, the world's largest medical library, it brings you information about diseases, conditions, and wellness issues in language you can understand. MedlinePlus offers reliable, up-to-date health information, anytime, anywhere, and for free. This is a trusted site and contains valuable information and can be accessed from a variety of different electronic devices.

A list of helpful websites can be found on www.JudithSands.com.

Software Tools/Applications

Many healthcare providers who have electronic medical records also have Patient Portals. These Patient Portals typically provide you access to a medication record that lists all the medication that the particular provider is aware that the individual is taking, vital signs, and various clinical reports (radiology and diagnostic studies, specialist consultations, lab work, etc.). Determine if your physicians have Patient Portals and get connected with the records. Ask your physician and hospice provider if they are using a specific mobile app to communicate with individuals and download it. Get connected to simplify the care management process.

There are also several free Health Information Technology applications that are available to assist with managing and securely sharing various types of health information. New apps are being frequently introduced. Explore what is available in the app store for a specific issue that you are tracking such as pain, digestion, depression, symptom management. The author does not endorse or recommend the value or utility of any app.

Before selecting any app, read and review information about each app to make independent and informed decisions about the value and helpfulness. Check out its compliance with HIPAA (information security) and reviews:

Apps to consider for organizing your medical records or creating a personal health record (there are many to consider):

CareSync has a number of options that help you in obtaining medical records, medication tracking & reminders and other features. Some portions of the app are free, and others have modest fees. ✎

Blue Button is a federal initiative that aims to make it easier for consumers to access their health records online. The iBlueButton app allows you to securely access and exchange electronic health records, including X-ray images and reports, lab results and visit summaries, with healthcare providers. ✎

Track My Medical Records is a handy, streamlined app that allows you to conveniently track your medical records, as well as those of your family members, and access them wherever you go. Data may be accessed offline, but it is backed up and stored in a cloud and transferred via encrypted connection for your security. There is also a website that can be used to access information from your desktop and other non-Android devices. ✎

FollowMyHealth Mobile provides smartphone access to a mobile version of their EHR. The app integrates with Apple Health to automatically update information such as blood pressure, changes in weight and glucose readings. FollowMyHealth also includes capabilities such as bill pay, prescription requests, appointment management and secure, two-way messaging with physicians. ✎

Medication Management Apps:

MedHelper Pill Reminder helps keep track of prescriptions, provides a medication alarm reminder, tracks scheduled doctor's appointments and men medications need to be reordered. Information can be shared with others. Available free for Android and Apple.

MedSimple is a medication resource center helps you find generic versions of your medications along with coupons and Patient Assistance Programs, provides medication reminders and detailed information about your medications. Available free for Android and Apple. ✎

MedCoach Medication Reminder helps to remind you to take medications as ordered, logs what was taken, connects to your pharmacy and provides drug information. Available free for Android and Apple.

Cancer.Net Mobile available in English and Spanish also features an interactive tool to keep track of questions to ask healthcare providers and record voice answers, a place to save information about prescribed medications, including photos of labels and bottles (on camera-enabled devices) and a symptom tracker to record the time and severity of symptoms and side effects. ✎

Glossary

Acute Care: Medical care administered usually in a hospital or by healthcare professionals for the treatment of a serious injury or illness.

Advance Care Planning (ACP): The discussion process using open communication, clarifying the individual's medical values, treatment/management goals and wishes with your physician and family. Can be started at any time and revisited periodically. Should be documented.

Advanced Directive (AD): Describes two types of legal documents, living wills and medical powers of attorney. These documents allow a person to give instructions about future medical care should the individual be unable to participate in medical decisions due to serious illness or incapacity. Each state regulates the use of advance directives differently.

Advanced Practice Registered Nurse (ARNP): also known as Advanced Practice Nurse or Nurse Practitioner, is a registered nurse who completes a graduate-level program and has additional clinical education, skills and responsibilities for administering patient care. Depending on the state, they may have prescribing authority and can practice independently and often work as physician extenders.

Artificial nutrition and hydration: Artificial nutrition and hydration supplements or replaces ordinary eating and drinking by giving a chemically balanced mix of nutrients and fluids through a tube placed directly into the stomach, the upper intestine or a vein.

Assisted living residence or "assisted living facility" (ALF): A long-term care living option providing personal care and support services including medication management, bathing, dressing, transportation and other practical day-to-day needs.

Bereavement: The unique individual grief experience of the bereaved person, through the anticipation of death and the subsequent adjustment to living following the death, of someone significant.

Brain death: The irreversible loss of all brain function. Most states legally define death to include brain death.

Capacity: In relation to end-of-life decision-making, an individual has medical decision-making capacity if he or she has the ability to understand the medical problem and the risks and benefits of the available treatment options. The individual's ability to understand other unrelated concepts is not relevant. The term is frequently used interchangeably with competency but is not the same. Competency is a legal status imposed by the court.

Cardiopulmonary resuscitation: Cardiopulmonary resuscitation (CPR) is a group of treatments used when someone's heart and/or breathing stops. CPR is used in an attempt to restart the heart and breathing. It may consist only of mouth-to-mouth breathing, or it can include pressing on the chest to mimic the heart's function and cause blood to circulate. Electric shock and drugs also are frequently used to stimulate the heart.

Certified nursing assistant (CNA): Provides basic care to individuals, assisting with activities of daily living (Bathing and Grooming, Dressing and Undressing, Meal Preparation and Feeding Functional Transfers, Safe Restroom Use and Maintaining Continence, Ambulation, Memory Care and Stimulation. CNA works under the direction of a nurse.

Chronic pain: Ongoing or recurrent pain lasting beyond the usual course of acute illness or injury or, generally, more than three to six months and adversely affecting the individual's well-being. A simpler definition of chronic or persistent pain is pain that continues when it should not.

Comfort Measures/Comfort Care: Medical care provided with the primary goal of keeping a person comfortable rather than prolonging life. Comfort measures are used to relieve pain and other symptoms.

Do Not Resuscitate (DNR)/Do Not Attempt Resuscitation (DNAR): A DNR order is a physician's written order instructing healthcare providers not to attempt cardiopulmonary resuscitation (CPR) in case of cardiac or respiratory arrest. A person with a valid DNR order will not be given CPR under these circumstances. Although the DNR order is written at the request of a person or surrogate, it must be signed by a physician to be valid. A non-hospital DNR order is written for individuals who are at home and do not want to receive CPR.

Doctor: The term generally refers to a person who has earned a Doctor of Medicine (MD), Doctor of Osteopathy (DO), Formally trained in medicine, treatment of disease through medication, medical procedure, and sometimes surgery.

Emergency Medical Services (EMS): A group of governmental and private agencies that provide emergency care, usually to persons outside of healthcare facilities; EMS personnel generally include paramedics, first responders, and other ambulance crew.

Euthanasia: The act or practice of killing or permitting the death of hopelessly sick or injured individuals (as persons or domestic animals) in a relatively painless way for reasons of mercy (Merriam-Webster, 2016a). Hospice is NOT Euthanasia.

Family: A family is defined as those closest to the individual in knowledge, care and affection who are connected through their common biological, legal, cultural, and emotional history.

Guardian: A court-appointed guardian or conservator having authority to make a healthcare decision for an individual.

Healthcare Proxy (Healthcare Agent, Durable Power of Attorney for Healthcare, Healthcare Power of Attorney, Medical Power of Attorney): The designated person named in an advance directive or as permitted under state law to make healthcare decisions on behalf of a person who is no longer able to make medical decisions.

Home Health/Healthcare Agency: Provides a wide range of healthcare services that can be given in your home for an illness or injury. Home healthcare is usually less expensive, more convenient, and just as effective as the care you get in a hospital or skilled nursing facility (SNF). Services include: Wound care for pressure sores or a surgical wound, Patient and caregiver education, Intravenous or nutrition therapy Injections, Monitoring serious illness and unstable health status.

Hospice: Hospice cares for the terminally ill individual in the last 6 months of life when the goal of care changes from cure to comfort. Hospice is a team approach to expert medical care, pain management, and emotional and spiritual support tailored to the person's needs and wishes. Most of the care is provided in the individual's home or the place they call home (nursing home, assisted living or independent living). When symptoms are acute and uncontrolled, hospice care may be provided in an inpatient care unit. The hospice benefit pays for all medical equipment and medication related to the terminal illness. The Hospice Benefit also cares for the family of the individual for 13 months after the death through grief counseling one on one or in groups. Medicare, Medicaid, TRICARE and most private insurances cover the cost of the Hospice Benefit. Counseling is free of charge. Considered to be the model for quality, compassionate care for people facing a life-limiting illness or injury, hospice, and palliative care involves a team-oriented approach to expert medical care, pain management, and emotional and spiritual support expressly tailored to the person's needs and wishes. Support is provided to the person's loved ones as well.

Inpatient hospice care: Care provided in an inpatient hospice unit or bed in a designated healthcare facility for a short period for intensive symptom management or at the very end-of-life when your loved one's condition cannot be managed at home.

Intravenous (IV) fluids: A small plastic tube (catheter) is inserted directly into the vein and fluids are given through the tube.

Intubation/Intubate: Placing a tube through the mouth or nose into the trachea (windpipe) to create and maintain an open airway to assist breathing tube to assist in breathing. Intubation is followed by mechanical ventilation.

Life-limiting Condition: A condition, illness or disease which:

a) Is progressive and fatal; and
b) The progress of which cannot be reversed by treatment

Life-sustaining treatment: Treatments (medical procedures) that replace or support an essential bodily function (may also be called life support treatments). Life-sustaining treatments include cardiopulmonary resuscitation, mechanical ventilation, artificial nutrition and hydration, dialysis, and other treatments.

Living Will: A type of advance directive in which a person documents (written or video) about the kinds of wishes (wants and does not want) about medical treatment under certain specific circumstances at the end-of-life and unable to communicate. It may also be called a "directive to physicians," "healthcare declaration," or "medical directive."

Long-term care (LTC): An array of healthcare, personal care, and social services generally provided over a sustained period of time to people of all ages with chronic conditions and with functional limitations. Their needs are met in a variety of care settings such as nursing homes, residential care facilities, or individual homes.

Medication Administration Record (MAR): A document used to record the list of medications prescribed and each time the medication was given to the individual.

Mechanical ventilation: Mechanical ventilation is used to support or replace the function of the lungs. A machine called a ventilator (or respirator) forces air into the lungs. The ventilator is attached to a tube inserted into the nose or mouth and down into the windpipe (or trachea).

Medical Futility/Medically Futile: The treatment is ineffective and does not follow commonly accepted community standards for treatment. It is inconsistent with the person's preferences or goals of care.

Medical Orders for Life-Sustaining Treatment - MOLST Form: A medical order form that tells others your wishes for life-sustaining treatments. The form is printed on bright pink paper so it can be easily identified in case of an emergency. MOLST forms are activated when you have a serious health condition.

Medical Orders for Life-Sustaining Treatment Program - MOLST Program: Improves the quality of medical care people receive at the end-of-life by turning individual goals and preferences into medical orders. It helps physicians, nurses, healthcare facilities and emergency personnel honor individual wishes regarding life-sustaining treatments.

Nurse: A person formally trained and licensed to provide care for the sick, disabled or dying, and who is skilled in promoting and maintaining health.

Patient-Centered Care: Healthcare that establishes a partnership among practitioners, individuals, and their families (when appropriate) to ensure that decisions respect individuals' wants, needs, and preferences and that individuals have the education and support they need to make decisions and participate in their own care.

Palliative care: A comprehensive treatment approach focusing on physical, psychological and spiritual needs of the individual. The goal is to achieve the best quality of life available to the individual by relieving suffering and controlling pain and symptoms. Care may be offered at any point during a chronic or terminal illness. One does not need to be in hospice to receive relief of symptoms of pain, nausea, shortness of breath, anorexia, fatigue and other symptoms due to illness. Palliative Care may be offered in the hospital or where the individual resides. Aims:

- Provides pain and symptom relief
- Affirms life and regards dying as a normal process

- Intends neither to hasten or postpone death
- Integrates psychological and spiritual care
- Offers a support system to live as actively as possible until death
- Offers a support system to assist family coping with the individual's illness and handle bereavement
- Uses a team to address the needs of the individual and families, including bereavement counseling
- Enhances the quality of life, and to positively influence the course of illness
- Applicable early in the course of illness, in conjunction with other therapies that are intended to prolong life, such as chemotherapy or radiation therapy, and includes those investigations needed to understand better and manage distressing clinical complications

Plan of Care: Provides direction (roadmap) for the individualized care of the individual; considering safety, collaboration, and condition and symptom management. A means for interdisciplinary (includes all the different specialties) communicating and organizing the care needed for an individual. It is based on a medical assessment (a review of the individual's conditions) initial and ongoing. It includes collaboration with the individual, family, and caregivers. It may include:

- The kinds of personal or healthcare services needed (including)
  - Washing or showering
  - Dressing changes
  - Pain management
  - Repositioning in bed
  - Spiritual
- What type of staff should provide these services
- Frequency of needed services
- Equipment or supplies needed (like a wheelchair or hospital bed)
- Diet and food preferences
- Individual or family wishes

Physician/Provider Orders for Life-Sustaining Treatment (POLST): An approach to improving end-of-life care in the United States, encouraging providers to speak with patients and create specific medical orders to be honored by health care workers during a medical crisis.

Power of attorney (POA): A legal document allowing one person to act in a legal matter on another's behalf regarding financial, real estate transactions, or medical decision making.

Respite care: Temporary, short-term relief and assistance for caregivers.

Respiratory arrest: The stopping of breathing. If breathing is not restored, an individual's heart eventually will stop beating, resulting in cardiac arrest.

Surrogate decision-making: Laws allow an individual or group of individuals (usually family members) to make decisions about medical treatments for an individual who has lost decision-making capacity and did not prepare an advance directive. A majority of states have passed statutes that permit surrogate decision making for individuals without advance directives.

Surrogate: A person who, by default, becomes the substitute decision-maker for an individual who has no appointed agent.

Tube-feeding: Providing fluids and/or nutrition by way of a tube placed into the stomach or intestines. On a short-term basis, the tube (Nasogastric tube or "NG-tube") is placed into the nose, down the throat, and into the stomach. For the long-term, the tube is placed directly into the stomach (Gastric, or "G-tube").

Unstable: The individual experiences the development of a new problem or rapid increase in the severity of existing problems, either of which requires an urgent change in management or sudden change in their situation requiring urgent intervention by a member of the care team.

Home Hospice Navigation

Ventilator: Also known as a respirator, is a machine that pushes air into the lungs through a tube placed in the trachea (breathing tube). Ventilators are used when a person cannot breathe on his or her own or cannot breathe effectively enough to provide adequate oxygen to the cells of the body or rid the body of carbon dioxide.

Withholding or withdrawing treatment: Stopping or discontinuing life-sustaining treatments them after they have been used for a certain period of time. Withholding is done when treatments are no longer helping to improve an individual's health, or the treatment is causing more symptoms.

Appendix A. Medication Administration Record

Name: _____				Physician: _____											Month & Year: _____													
Medication	**Hour**	1	2	3	4	5	6	7	8	9	10	11	12	13	14	15	16	17	18	19	20	21	22	23	24	25	26	27	28	29	30	31

R = Refused   **D** = Discontinued   **C** = Changed

Remember to Record at Time of Administration

Appendix B.   Home Health Agency Checklist

Use this checklist when choosing a home health agency.

Name of the home health agency _____

Question	Yes/No	Comments
1. Medicare-certified?		
2. Medicaid-certified (if you have both Medicare and Medicaid)?		
3. Offers the specific health care services I need (like skilled nursing services or physical therapy)?		
4. Meets my special needs (like language or cultural preferences)?		
5. Offers the personal care services I need (like help bathing, dressing, and using the bathroom)?		
6. Offers the support services I need, or can help me arrange for additional services, like Meals on Wheels, that I may need?		
7. Has staff that can provide the type and hours of care my doctor ordered and start when I need them?		
8. Is recommended by my hospital discharge planner, doctor, or social worker?		
9. Has staff available at night and on weekends for emergencies?		
10. Explained what my insurance will cover and what I must pay out-of-pocket?		
11. Does background checks on all staff?		
12. Has letters from satisfied patients, family members, and doctors that testify to the home health agency providing good care?		

https://www.medicare.gov/what-medicare-covers/home-health-care/Home%20Health%20Agency%20Checklist.pdf

Visit Home Health Compare at www.medicare.gov/homehealthcompare for more information

Appendix C.   Funeral Pricing Checklist

Make copies of this tool and check with several funeral homes to compare costs.

	Facility 1	Facility 2	Facility 3
"Simple" disposition of the remains			
Immediate burial			
Immediate cremation			
If the cremation process is extra, how much is it?			
Donation of the body to a medical school or hospital			
"Traditional," full-service burial or cremation			
Basic services fee for the funeral director and staff			
Pickup of body			
Embalming			
Other preparation of body			
Least expensive casket			
Description, including model #			
Outer Burial Container (vault)			
Description			
Visitation/viewing — staff and facilities			
Funeral or memorial service — staff and facilities			
Graveside service, including staff and equipment			
Hearse			
Other vehicles			
Other Services			
Forwarding body to another funeral home			
Receiving body from another funeral home			
Cemetery/Mausoleum Costs			
Cost of lot or crypt (if you don't already own one)			
Perpetual care			
Opening and closing the grave or crypt			
Grave liner, if required			
Marker/monument (including setup)			
There may be additional costs based on religious obligations including			
A shroud			
Religious articles necessary for the service			
Additional visitation hours			
Storage fees / delaying the burial			
Weekend or afterhours burials			

Appendix D.   Contact Information

Keep track of the hospice team members working with you and when visits are planned.

- Hospice Name and Contact information: _____

- Nurse:_____

- Aide/CNA: _____

- Social Worker: _____

- Spiritual Care: _____

- Other: _____

- Copies of Advance Directives (Living Wills / DNR / DNAR / Durable Power of Attorney for Healthcare Decisions) should be kept readily available in the home and not stored in safe-deposit boxes. Copies should be given to physicians, local hospitals, independent and Assisted Living Facility (ALF) management staff.
    - If there is a living will; what is designated?
    - Original document location / who has access?
    - Where are copies located?
- Are there any religious practices that need to address?
    - Clergy contact information
    - Is clergy aware?
    - Who will contact the clergy?

Appendix E.   Caregiver Communication

Use this as a guide when there is a handoff between caregivers. The communication between caregivers should be **clear**, **concise**, and **factual**.

Personal Care

- Any issues with discomfort, toileting, bathing, repositioning or turning
- Share any skin redness, bowel movements (constipation or diarrhea), and urination (issues with passing water)
- Any issues with dressing, walking or movement

Medication

- Intolerance of routine medication
- Review the Medication Administration List (MAR)
    - Noting last doses of medications given
    - Need for pain or symptom management medications
- Breakthrough pain or uncontrolled symptoms

Food & Nutrition

- Amount and type of food and liquids taken
- Difficulty eating or swallowing
- Requests for special foods or foods to be limited

Any other issues

- Caregiver concerns
- Visitor encouragement or restriction
- Special requests

Made in the USA
Monee, IL
26 October 2023

45280575R00066